D0869108

Reasonably Raw

Reasonably Raw

Eating Your Way to Health, Happiness,
& Wholeness

Dr. Frank J. Ferendo

PROCESS PUBLISHING COMPANY
WESTERLY, RHODE ISLAND

Copyright © 2008 by Frank Ferendo

All rights reserved. No part of this publication may be reproduced, stored in a retrieval system or transmitted in any form or by any means, electronic, mechanical, photocopying, recording, or otherwise without prior written permission of the copyright holder, except brief quotations.

Disclaimer: This publication contains the ideas and opinions of the author. It is intended to provide helpful information only. The book is not intended as medical advice. The author disclaims any responsibility for liability or loss incurred as a result of the use and application of the contents of this book.

Published by   Cover and book design by
Process Publishing Company   Jill Shorrock
10 Sunny Dr.
Westerly, R.I. 02891

Library of Congress Cataloging-in-Publication Data

Ferendo, Frank
Reasonably Raw: Eating Your Way to Health, Happiness, and Wholeness
By Dr. Frank J. Ferendo
p. cm.

ISBN-978-0-9795180-2-7

LCCN: 2008933869

Library of Congress subject heading:
    1. Raw food diet. 2. Raw foods. I. Title.

The author may be contacted at fjferendo@cox.net.
Videos for recipes and inspiration may be accessed at reasonablyraw.blogspot.com.
More information may be found at frankferendo.com.

Printed in the United States of America

This book is dedicated to my children:

Gina—the inspiration for this book and so much more.

Frankie—creative passionate wild genius.

Angela—so much like her dad.

You are the true loves of my life and my precious teachers!

ACKNOWLEDGMENTS

I would like to thank Gina and Steven Law
for getting me started on the raw food journey
and keeping me inspired.
I would like to thank Frankie and Angela
for their inspiration—
and you too, Megan and Andy.
I would like to thank my editor Cherie Gingerich
and book and cover designer Jill Shorrock.

CONTENTS

PREFACE

I'd like to share with you some things I've learned over the past several years that are quite amazing and can bring you much happiness and health. What I have learned has so changed my life that I am extremely excited to be sharing it with you. The ideas in this book can make you healthier and happier than you ever thought possible.

Much of what we believe about food is wrong. Our ideas of what is good and bad for us come from corporations that benefit financially from our eating their foods and not eating others. We have been *taught* (brainwashed is more accurate) by these companies since the 1940's, when it was first discovered that eating animals was maybe not such a good thing. Ever since then, the food industries have used all their power and resources to convince us otherwise.

You should know that from scientific research (unbiased research) we now know that eating cooked foods causes our stomachs and intestines to have coatings of thick mucus to protect against toxins and acids. Our pancreases have become about twice the size of that of a horse. When we eat cooked foods, our body thinks it has an infection and begins making white blood cells.

Cooked food fiber passes slowly through our digestive system and partially rots, ferments, and putrefies. Our bodies work hard and get little. Cooking destroys the nutrients in foods. But you probably already know that. Raw foods contain enzymes that survive the hydrochloric acid of the stomach and enter our blood and organs. These enzymes act as catalysts to feed our cells, along with the organic vitamins, minerals, proteins, and fats found in uncooked foods.

I have purposely kept this book short. I've waded through many books and articles, weeded out the extra verbiage, and written down the essential facts and truths about healthful cultures around the world, the food industry, and the raw vegan diet. I have included what I felt was the best of the best and what works.

While keeping this book short, I have added much more information on my website. You can also go to my **youtube** channel, www.youtube.com/user/frankferendo, and see how to make many of the recipes in the book. You can visit my website, frankferendo.com, and find much more information and many more resources. In addition, just google "raw foods" and you will find many more helpful websites, blogs, newsletters, and discussion groups. I highly recommend using **youtube** to find plenty of interesting raw food recipe demonstrations. They will inspire you!

Becoming more aware of how your food and diet beliefs have been carefully cultivated by the food industry will open you up to the possibility that there may be a better way to eat. Becoming more aware of how good you can feel eating more raw foods may inspire you to give it a try. And seeing how easy it is to gradually add raw foods to your life, as demonstrated by the videos, you will be glad that you took the time to consider being reasonably raw.

INTRODUCTION

"Take care of your body with steadfast fidelity. The soul must see through these eyes alone, and if they are dim, the whole world is clouded."

—JOHANN WOLFGANG VON GOETHE

I am not sure how or why I became interested in healthy living. My upbringing would not have suggested it. The only thing that comes to mind is that it must have been through reading some book or magazine. And then during college I began a daily running routine. The first time I ran, barely making a mile, I came home coughing, wheezing, and coughing up phlegm.

Several years later, in 1977, Jim Fixx's *The Complete Book of Running* came out and I got serious about exercise. Eventually I worked up to my current practice of jogging five miles a day. I've since added some weight training.

My first experiments in improving my diet involved making a breakfast drink of brewer's yeast and milk. In 1987 the book *Fit For Life* by Harvey and Marilyn Diamond became a best seller. Based on the principles of *Natural Hygiene*, which is one of the raw food branches covered in this book, the Diamonds encouraged people to eat lots of fruit on an empty stomach, as well as eating live high-water content foods, along with proper food combining (an example would be not eating a protein and a carbohydrate together in one meal). I read the Diamonds' book and tried to follow its teachings. The end result was that ever since then I have always eaten fruit for breakfast.

Two years later, the Juiceman, Jay Kordich, came through town telling his story of how juicing raw fruits and vegetables saved him from cancer. I heard him on the radio and promptly bought a juice machine. I didn't stop at one juicer; I kept buying them until I was convinced I had the best one. I juiced carrots everyday for about ten years. (I also forced carrot juice on my kids, with uncertain results, although all three are health-conscious now and my oldest daughter makes juices for my grandchildren.)

I was getting the message about health everywhere I turned. Then in the late 80's I met a woman well beyond seventy years old. She looked years younger and told me of her thirty-year-old boyfriend who could not keep up with her. She said that yoga was her secret. So I started doing yoga. She also told me to read John Robbins's *Diet for a New America*. The book tells of the horrors of the meat and dairy industry and advocates a vegan diet.

So convincing was the book that I became a vegetarian for one year. My daughter Gina became one permanently. I desperately wanted to stop eating animals and dairy products, but I did not have the will power. I felt guilty about the slaughtering of animals, but my desire for hamburgers was greater. I knew that the animal food industry was a significant polluter of our environment. Still, I couldn't make myself change my diet.

"Transformation is through the body, not away from it."

—ECKHART TOLLE

For nearly twenty years I did not make any more health changes. I ran every day, I ate my fruits and vegetables, I was very conscious of what I put into my mouth. I should have been very healthy. I was doing much better than the average American, I thought. And then I went for a physical and the doctor told me, practically with glee in his voice, that my cholesterol was 242.

How could this be? "Doc, I eat healthy foods; I run." To which he replied, "It's probably your genes. If you can't get your cholesterol down by changing your diet, we'll have to put you on Lipitor."

You have got to be kidding me! I am not taking a pill. There is no way I am going on a drug. Putting a foreign substance into my body is not natural. Lipitor may make my cholesterol level go down, but will it make me healthier? If I don't change my diet, have I really made things better or have I just masked the problem? It seems to me that drug companies make a lot of money, and all one gets is the false sense of security that you have done something when in reality that isn't the case. Eliminating the symptom doesn't get rid of the cause.

Meanwhile, my vegetarian daughter Gina informed me that she

and her husband were "going raw."

"What do you mean? You're not eating cooked foods anymore? Gina, I've always admired you for not eating meat, but this is crazy. What will you eat?" I forget what she said, but I walked away thinking that she had gone too far. I knew I shouldn't have made her drink carrot juice.

A month later I saw her and my son-in-law Stephen—they were literally glowing. I could not believe it. They were radiating health. Now I was interested. I asked her for a book on this raw food stuff (of course, I need a book) and she gave me Victoria Boutenko's *Green for Life*. I read the book, fooled around for a bit with green smoothies and salads, but then gave it up. I could not stop eating hamburgers and French fries, pizza, ice cream, and you name it. I'll live with the high cholesterol. I run five miles a day, there is no way I can have heart disease, I thought. I decided to take my chances—but the seed had been planted.

In the spring of 2007 I came down with a cold that just wouldn't go away. Finally I went to a doctor for an antibiotic to put an end to it. The nurse took my blood pressure. "Your blood pressure is 160 over 100." She tried my other arm. Just as bad. Now I have high blood pressure along with the cholesterol.

That was it. There was no longer any denying that, given all that I was doing for my health, I still had problems. Since I refused to start taking pills, I decided I had to do something. I began reading and everything I read pointed to "going raw."

In the beginning it wasn't even about being raw that got me thinking and motivated. Three books ended up on my desk. They were about how to make changes, how the food industry in America works, and the ethics of eating animals. So before I even began the process of trying to eat raw foods, the universe, in all its wisdom, gave me a few tools to turn away from a cooked, animal-based diet and taught me about how to go about making these changes.

Changing For Good by James Prochaska, John Norcross, and Carlo Diclemente explained to me that change is a process; it does not come all at once through will power. There are stages of change. We move little by little. Change involves consciousness-raising, finding alternatives to old behaviors, expressing and accessing feelings and emotions, taking action, enjoying the rewards of change, and helping relationships. There is a *reasonable* way to go about making changes.

And then I found myself reading Michael Pollan's bestseller *The Omnivore's Dilemma.* Here I discovered how many of our food attitudes and beliefs are controlled and influenced by big business interests. We as a country are suffering from a national eating disorder, and it is fueled by the marketing of corporations and their influence over the legislative process through lobbyists. We don't eat what we would naturally eat, we eat what we have been manipulated into eating.

The book that kicked me over the edge into action was *The Way We Eat: Why Our Food Choices Matter* by Peter Singer and Jim Mason. I was confronted with the impact of my food choices and how they affected people, animals, and the planet. Singer and Mason describe the incredible cruelty that factory farming inflicts on the animals we eat. They reveal the lengths that the food industry goes to hide what actually goes on in those farms. Most alarming of all was the destruction to the environment caused by the food industry and the amount of natural resources consumed. (If Americans gave up eating animals, the oil saved would be like taking every car in America off the road.) By this time, my emotions had joined what I knew in my head. I was ready to change.

Now I was ready to begin reading and experimenting with the raw food diet. I did more than experiment; I used the skills that I acquired in getting my doctorate to research what was out there on becoming a "raw fooder." There are numerous people promoting various programs for eating a raw, living-foods diet, and many of them don't agree with each other on what is best. I soon found that I needed to determine who was helpful and who wasn't. I needed to find out what was scientifically based and what was just self-promotion and marketing.

I read everything I could get my hands on. To me, this was a life and death situation. I wanted the truth. I wanted to discount what was motivated by what people were selling; and people do have products to sell even in the raw food movement. I went to the Raw Spirit Festival in Sedona, Arizona and saw firsthand enough marketing and contradictory approaches to health to make my head hurt. (I had to escape and have a burger late at night when no one was looking!)

Ultimately, I felt I had to write a book so that I could put all that I learned in one place and get my thoughts around what the best approach to getting my health back was. I am totally convinced that eating raw food is the way to go. Does that mean going 100 percent as most advocate? That is something you have to decide for yourself. I've tried to assemble the best of what is out there in this book. And I've tried to point out the best that each person has to offer. The answers to life's challenges are not black and white. I think an eclectic approach works best; why not take what makes sense to you from everything that is out there? That is what I have done here. I've tried to find the common thread that runs through all the approaches to raw food. I hope it works for you.

This book is the result of what I found out as I made a serious commitment to change my diet, to change my thoughts about food, and to change my mind about what it is to live a healthy life. In the following chapters I take information from all the many books I read and all the experimenting I did and try to give to you a simple guide to beginning a raw food journey. I've tried to inspire and motivate so you don't have to one day be on your deathbed saying, "Geez, I really wish I had taken better care of myself."

Eating more raw foods can save your life, give you more energy than you ever dreamed, and if you learn how to make some of the cacao recipes, you will certainly smile a whole lot more than you ever did. I know I do.

Books to Get You Motivated:

The Way We Eat: Why Our Food Choices Matter, by Peter Singer and Jim Mason. 2006. Rodale (Holtzbrinck Publishers).

Eat to Live: The Revolutionary Formula for Fast and Sustained Weight Loss, by Joel Fuhrman, M.D. 2003. Little, Brown and Company.

The Food Revolution: How Your Diet Can Help Save Your Life and Our World, by John Robbins. 2001. Conari Press.

The Omnivore's Dilemma: A Natural History of Four Meals, by Michael Pollan. 2006. The Penguin Press.

Chapter 1

The Long-Living People

*"How would you like to live in a land where cancer has not
yet been invented? A land where an optometrist discovers to
his amazement that everyone has perfect 20-20 vision? A land
where cardiologists cannot find a single trace of coronary
heart disease? How would you like to live in a land where no
one ever gets ulcers, appendicitis or gout? A land where men
of 80 and 90 father children, and there's nothing unusual
about men and women enjoying vigorous life at the age of
100 or 120?"*

—JANE KINDERLEHRER

Considering the natural diets of our closest relatives in the wild, the
primates, is one way to think about what we would eat if we were not
influenced by culture or people selling a product for profit. It seems
logical that a natural diet would be best. We will explore that in several
chapters, but for now I'd like to look at people and societies that live
the longest and have the healthiest lives.

In the next two chapters we will do exactly that. First we look at
four cultures where people live to be extremely old and healthy at the
same time. Then we will examine one of the largest studies concerning
the relation of diet to health ever conducted—the China Study.

The Abkhasians

In the Caucasus Mountains of southern Russia live the Abkhasians. In the 1960's the Soviets made claims that the people there were living to be well into their 100's. One Abkhasian got his picture on a postage stamp for being 168 years old. The Dannon yogurt company went out there and made a popular commercial featuring a 110-year-old mother telling her 89-year-old son to eat his yogurt.

It turns out that these people were not as old as they claimed. They were probably "only" in their 90's and early 100's. More important than their years was their physical fitness and mental alertness. Researchers found them to be enjoying extremely good health. Only the very oldest had wrinkles. Few needed glasses and most still had their own teeth.

What was their secret? How did they keep healthy into old age? The Abkhasians get a lot of exercise living in the mountains. There is no question that physical activity is essential. They maintained their physical fitness into old age by not retiring and working in the orchards and gardens.

The other factor contributing to their health is diet. Breakfast consists of fresh salad, cornmeal porridge, and a fermented drink made from goat's milk. Between meals they eat a great deal of fruit. Nuts are also an important part of their diet. They eat almost no meat. They do not eat fatty foods, sugar, salt, or butter. Overeating is considered socially inappropriate.

The Abkhasians do not eat yogurt despite the Dannon commercials.

The average cholesterol level of those over age 100 is below 100. There is one more thing that may contribute to their long productive lives— the elders are respected and revered simply for being old.

The Vilcabambans

Three hundred miles to the south of Quito, Ecuador, high in the Andes mountains, is the village of Vilcabamba; it is also called the Valley of Longevity. Here the inhabitants frequently live into their 100's with youthful vigor and vitality. Degenerative diseases do not exist there. No cancer, no diabetes, no osteoporosis, no Alzheimer's. No heart disease or high blood pressure.

International scientists have studied the Vilcabambanas for half a century and the conclusion has been that their health is the result of their diet and high levels of physical activity. There are no supermarkets in Vilcabamba, no processed foods. Vegetables and fruits are picked fresh daily and eaten on the spot. Occasionally they have milk or eggs, but their diet is essentially fruits, vegetables, seeds, nuts, beans, and whole grains.

It is interesting to note that their protein comes from vegetables, whole grains, and beans. Their fat comes from avocados, seeds, and nuts. They do not consume a large amount of calories compared to American standards. Overweight people cannot be found in Vilcabamba. Because of where they live, fresh fruit and vegetables are available year round.

The Hunza

Twenty thousand feet up in the Himalayan Mountains in northwestern Pakistan is Hunza. Probably the most famous of all for being a place where the people live well past 100 and where they have perfect eyesight, no cancer, no heart disease, and no crime. (Also, no money, no banks, no taxes, and no stores.)

It isn't that these people just are not sickly, they are strong and active their whole lives. They swim in ice-covered streams, they build retaining walls for their gardens; they play wild games of volleyball and polo. What makes them so healthy?

A look at their diet shows that it is quite different from what we have been told is necessary for health by the food industry and our government. They eat less than half the protein and a third of the fat that we do. And it all comes from fruits, vegetables, and grains. They do not eat animals. No food is processed and it is all fresh. The closest they come to processing is drying their fruits. They have a law against spraying their gardens with pesticide.

The Hunzas eat a lot of apricots, and a lot of sprouts. Served at every meal is their bread called "chappti." They call it a bread, but it is not really baked. After grinding fresh wheat, barley, or millet, they knead it with only water, no yeast, and then place it on a grill for a moment, just long enough to warm it.

The Hunzas and the other long-living people didn't eat a mostly raw vegetarian diet because they wanted to—they didn't really have a choice. High up in the mountains there isn't a lot of wood for cooking and food to keep animals. So, they mostly eat plants and eat them raw.

It isn't just that these people live to be old, it's that they are disease-free that is most impressive. The old do not suffer from fatigue, poor eyesight, high blood pressure, or obesity. Very much like the people of Abkhasia and Vilcabamba.

Besides extraordinary good health their diets are quite similar. Approximately 70% of their calories come from carbohydrates (in the form of fresh fruits, vegetables, and whole grains), 20% from fat (from nuts and seeds), and 10% from protein. The Abkhasia include about 10% animal products, but the Vilcabamba and Hunza only 1%. Almost no salt is used and there is no use of sugar or processed food.

Okinawa

Birth records have been meticulously kept in Okinawa since 1879. So the ages of these long-lived people on this southernmost Japanese island chain are not disputable. Every city and town has a family register dating back well over a hundred years. And since 1975 the Japan government has been studying the health and longevity of these people.

There are 800 centenarians out of a population of 1.3 million. The Okinawans do not retire. Is this what keeps them healthy, or do they not retire because they are so healthy? According to researchers there are four reasons for their extraordinary well being. Social support, psycho-spiritual attitudes, diet, and exercise.

Until relatively recently Okinawa was a separate country from Japan and evolved with a different culture, diet, and religious beliefs.

And their incidence of disease is also different from Japan (and the West). Like the Abkhasians, Vilcabambans, and the Hunza, heart disease, cancer, diabetes, and other diseases are rare among these people.

The Okinawan diet consists of a lot of sweet potato, green leafy vegetables, and protein from soy foods such as tofu and miso. They do eat fish. But diet alone is not the secret to their success. They get a good night's sleep. That may be related to what they eat because it is hard to sleep well when your stomach is busy digesting a heavy meal. The Okinawans also have a strong sense of responsibility and hold themselves accountable for their lives.

Probably more than anything, and similar to the other long-lived people in this chapter is that the Okinawans do not consume a lot of calories compared to the standard American diet. By consuming mostly fruits, vegetables, and grains, they get the nutrition they need without the calories.

Living Long

Maybe we could learn something from people who live long, active, disease-free lives. It only makes sense to pay attention to others who are succeeding at something. In this case it is something near and dear to all of us—our health.

It seems to me that exercise and working outdoors is primary. Eating a plant-based diet is also essential. Having some kind of spiritual practice is important. And staying connected to other people is also important. None of these alone is sufficient. All of the long-lived peoples of the world incorporate all of these components into their lives. A life-style based on these principles, and not on those of advertisers and promoters, would surely be an improvement for all of us.

Additional Reading on the Long-Living People

Healthy at 100: How You Can—at any age—Dramatically Increase Your Life Span and Your Health Span by John Robbins. 2007. Ballantine Books.

Chapter 2

The China Study

"...the Grand Prix of all epidemiological studies...the most comprehensive large study ever undertaken of the relationship between diet and the risk of developing disease."

—THE NEW YORK TIMES

He began his career as a researcher at MIT promoting better health through eating more meat, eggs, and milk. Growing up on a farm, he believed that high quality animal protein was necessary for good health. But later on, while researching why so many Filipino children were getting liver cancer, Dr. T. Colin Campbell discovered that the children who ate the most protein were the ones contracting the cancer.

Campbell became involved in a twenty-year research project, a partnership between Cornell University, Oxford University, and the Chinese Academy of Preventive Medicine, and the results became known as the China Study. The study researched the connection between diseases and lifestyle factors in rural China and Taiwan. As the New York Times article states, it is "the most comprehensive large study ever undertaken of the relationship between diet and the risk of developing disease."

The findings were startling, more than 8,000 statistically significant associations between diet and disease. The people who ate the most animal-based foods got the most disease. The people who ate the most plant-based foods got the least. **The most important finding out of Dr. Campbell's research is that the greatest threat to good health is animal protein.** It's not fat, it's not carbohydrates, it's animal protein. That includes chicken and fish and dairy.

The China Project

The China Project studied the death rates from twelve different kinds of cancer in more than 2,400 counties, and 880 million citizens, comprising nearly 96 percent of the population of those counties. More than 650,000 people worked on the project, the largest ever of its kind. The results showed massive variations in the cancer rates among the different counties. What makes this study so significant is that those being studied came from similar genetic backgrounds. This suggests that cancer is caused by lifestyle and environmental factors and not genetics. In some cases cancers were found to be 100 times greater in one county compared to another.

What makes this study so useful is that within China there are wide ranges of diets. It is unique because diet as studied in the West usually involves the contrast between those rich in animal-based foods and those very rich. In China many diets include mostly plant-based foods. This led to comparing incidence of disease in China to the West.

People in the study were chosen from rural and semi-rural parts of

China in order to be assured that the participants lived in the same area for most of their lives.

Blood Cholesterol

A comparison of the prevalence of cancers, heart disease, and diabetes in each county studied in China with lifestyle and diet indicated that blood cholesterol is linked to these diseases with more than a 99 percent certainty. Lower blood cholesterol levels indicate lower rates of cancer and heart disease.

What was very interesting was that low cholesterol in China is not what we think of in America. In America we are told to keep it below 200. The average level in China was below 130. In some areas women had cholesterol levels of below 90.

Other studies show that the consumption of animal protein increases blood cholesterol. We have been told that saturated fat and dietary cholesterol, raise cholesterol levels, which is true, but animal protein is even more effective at doing the job. You think you are eating healthy by eating lean chicken. It's the protein that is responsible for cholesterol more than the fat.

Protein

Protein, yes, we all need lots of protein to build strong bodies. That's what we've been told. It is interesting that when the human body is at its most active stage of growth, the first several years, it is feeding naturally on breast milk. The protein percentage of breast milk is about 7 percent. Only 7 percent of a baby's diet consists of protein. The typical American diet contains three times as much.

If a baby doesn't need all that protein, why do adults? The answer probably does not have anything to do with good health. I believe that we have been brainwashed and conditioned to think we need huge amounts of protein our entire lives.

Let's go back to Dr. Campbell's work. While trying to find out why the more wealthy children in the Philippines were getting cancer and the poorer were not, he came across an Indian research paper that pointed to protein as being the answer. Laboratory rats, predisposed to get liver cancer by being given aflatoxin, when fed a diet of 20 percent protein; all developed cancer. Those rats fed a diet of 5 percent protein developed not one case. This led Dr. Campbell to examine more closely the diets of the Filipino children. It turns out that the more "wellfed" children consumed considerably more protein than their poorer counterparts.

Cancer and Protein

To get a better understanding of this, let's look at how cancer develops. Cancer grows like a lawn. First the seeds get planted, then they sprout and mature, and then they spread and go wild. When we ingest carcinogens we plant the seeds of cancer. Carcinogens mutate healthy cells into cancer-prone cells. The seeds are there in our bodies ready to germinate. That in itself does no damage to the body and goes on all the time.

The germination stage can last a long time. In fact, without the right conditions, the cancer will not ever sprout. Just as grass seeds need water and warmth to grow, cancer also needs the right ingredients. It is also known that, like in the growth of a lawn, if the right conditions are removed, the growth can be stopped. This is critical to our understanding of cancer and how to prevent its taking hold.

If the favorable conditions persist we have cancer cell growth spreading out of control, creating tumors and moving to other tissues in the body. What does all this have to do with protein? Funded by the National Institutes of Health (NIH), the American Cancer Society, and the American Institute for Cancer Research, Campbell and others have spent the last twenty years studying cancer and nutrition. This is what they found:

Protein creates the conditions for the germination of the cancer seeds by increasing enzyme activity that allows carcinogens to bind to and mutate DNA. Campbell and his associates found that low protein diets protected against cancer growth by allowing fewer carcinogens into cells. Furthermore, **low protein diets actually reduced tumors.**

Cell clusters that are precursors to tumor development, called foci, are entirely dependent upon protein to grow. Even the consumption of carcinogens did not result in tumors unless there was sufficient protein. In their tests with rats, carcinogenic foci did not develop until protein levels reached 10 percent. Above that level tumor development took off. Below that level not one rat developed cancer.

Further studies showed that not all proteins had the same effect on the cancerous cells. Plant protein, even at high levels, did not promote growth. Protein from cow's milk, however, was the worst. Why have we not heard of this until now? I would suspect that the cattle and dairy lobbyists are doing their job.

Fats and Cancer

In America we consume more than 35 percent of our calories from fat. Scientists have been saying that this is too much. But they haven't pushed to go much below the 30 percent figure. Studies show a close correlation between fat intake and breast cancer. The China Study disclosed that fat consumption varied between 6 and 24 percent of calories from fat. And even at that level there was a significant reduction in risk at the lower levels. In other words, to be protected from risks of cancer, dietary fat needs to be down to around 10 percent. Dr. Doug Graham, a proponent of raw food, teaches in his books that a healthy diet consists of 80 percent carbohydrates, 10 percent protein, and 10 percent fats. We will be discussing this in a later chapter.

Diet

So where does all of this leave us? Quite simply: the food we eat and our nutrition play a very big role in the triggering of disease. Plant-based foods lower blood cholesterol. Lower blood cholesterol is related to lower rates of disease. Animal based foods increase blood cholesterol. Higher blood cholesterol is related to higher rates of disease.

What the China Study points out is that it is not enough to simply eat more fruits and vegetables…and keep eating our burgers, and chicken, and steaks, and salmon. A salad before a meal and bowl of fruit for desert does not begin scratch the surface. In order to enjoy the protection of good nutrition there needs to be a radical change. Even a little animal protein can trigger cancer in humans. Blood cholesterol has to be drastically lowered to prevent heart disease. Protein has to be reduced to prevent cancer.

Fat and cholesterol are factors in all kinds of illness, but what we miss in all of this is that **it is the animal protein that we bring into our bodies that cause fat and cholesterol to be there in the first place.** The meat and dairy industries want us to think we can lower our fat and cholesterol and eat their products at the same time. That just is not possible. All the lean hamburger, lean chicken, and lean fish in the world is not going to protect you. The problem isn't in the fat; it's in the protein. The lesson of the China study suggests that we need to eliminate protein from our diets. We have to stop eating animals.

By the way, plant protein and plant fat, are good for you. In fact, they lower your risks of heart disease and cancer. It is also interesting that the Chinese in the study, consuming a plant-based diet, were ingesting more calories per pound of body weight than us Americans— and they are slimmer. Why? Because a plant-based diet allows the body to burn calories as body heat instead of storing them as body fat as do the calories from an animal-based diet. In addition, carbohydrates from plants provide more energy fuel than a more heavy and fatty food from animals. It is no wonder that when you read about people turning to a more live food way of eating they proclaim they have so much more energy, need less sleep, have fewer aches and pains—the human body likes the lightness of a plant-based diet.

Principles of Good Health

In summary, Dr. Campbell promotes eight principles for good health as a result of his years of scientific research:

1. The nutrients in food are packaged together, they work in concert; it is too simplistic to think that one specific nutrient by itself will provide a benefit.
2. That is why supplements will not save you. Isolating nutrients will not provide the benefits that whole foods provide.
3. Plants provide all their nutrients in a more absorbable and useful way than animals.
4. Research shows that genes do not determine disease alone. In most cases it takes poor environment and diet to express and trigger them.
5. Nutrition trumps toxic chemicals. Cancer causing chemicals are all around us. But research shows that nutrition determines if the chemicals cause disease.
6. Nutrition can halt or reverse disease in its later stages.
7. Good nutrition supports health across the board.

8. Good health is a holistic undertaking: it requires exercise, the caring for emotional and mental needs, and concern for the places where we live.

To learn more about The China Study:

The China Study: Startling Implications for Diet, Weight Loss and Long- Term Health, by Campbell, T. Colin, Ph.D. and Campbell, Thomas M. II. (2004) Benbella Books.

Chapter 3

Victoria Boutenko and Green Smoothies

"Even if you are eating Snickers and Mountain Dew…you can still benefit from a green smoothie…get on board!"

—FROM *THE HAPPY FOODY BLOG*

My daughter Gina and son-in-law Steven had been eating raw for several months and I had seen the difference it was making in their health. I asked Gina to recommend a book to get me started and she suggested two books by Victoria Boutenko, *12 Steps to Raw Foods* and *Green For Life*. The *Green For Life* book was shorter and had a more interesting cover so I chose that one. Plus I wasn't really trying to step into raw foods. It turns out that that book was the ideal place for me to begin.

Green For Life by Boutenko is not about giving up cooked foods and only eating raw; it is not about giving up anything, only adding green smoothies to one's daily diet. While I wanted to get healthy, as were my children, I did not want to give up my hamburgers and french fries.

Boutenko and her family started eating raw foods back in 1993 when they all were experiencing major health problems at the same time. Victoria herself weighted 280 pounds and suffered from arrhythmia (irregular heartbeat). Her husband had hyperthyroidism, rheumatoid arthritis, and a constant heartbeat of more than 140. Her daughter Valya had asthma and allergies. And her son Sergei was just diagnosed with diabetes. It was the thought of insulin shots and the eventual side-effects (kidney and eyesight failure) that pushed Victoria over the edge. She searched everywhere for an alternative for her son.

Several months later she found out about raw foods from a woman who claimed to be cured of cancer twenty years ago by changing her diet. This was enough for Victoria and after overcoming her husband's initial resistance (he refused to give up eating his meat and potatoes until his doctors told him that he needed to have his thyroid removed, otherwise he would die—he decided to try raw foods instead) she threw out all of their cooked and processed food and the whole family ate only raw food from then on.

Obviously it was not easy going cold turkey, but the seriousness of their illnesses was a great motivator and they have continued to eat only raw food ever since. Victoria has written several books about her family's experience, all of which I highly recommend. Which brings us back to *Green For Life*.

While eating raw foods is a good thing, it is not easy to transition into, of course, unless you and your family are facing life and death health issues. Most of us are not motivated enough to give up the foods we have enjoyed all our lives. While I certainly wanted to enjoy the health that I was seeing my daughter achieve, I did not want to change my diet all that much. And that is why I feel that I was fortunate to begin my raw food journey with the *Green For Life* book.

Green For Life is not about giving up anything. It is about making one simple addition to your diet—a green smoothie. The Boutenko family had been eating raw for about ten years, but they began to experience a plateau. While their old illnesses never returned, they felt that they could be healthier.

Victoria began researching ways to improve their diet even more. She wanted to find out if there was anything missing from her raw diet that could make a difference. Her search led her to investigate the eating habits of our closest relatives in the animal kingdom. Chimpanzees share more than 99 percent of our DNA sequence. Believing that humans have lost their natural way of eating, maybe chimpanzees could point her back in the right direction.

It turns out that a chimp diet in the wild consists of roughly 50 percent fruits, 40 percent greens, 7 percent seeds, nuts, pith, and bark, and about 3 percent insects. This was not how the Boutenko family and most other raw foodists were eating (particularly the insects). Many people in the raw food movement tend to eat fewer greens and more nuts, seeds, and oils.

Boutenko also discovered that chimpanzees mostly feed on fruit in the morning, take a nap or play, then eat mostly greens in the afternoon. They stop eating for the day by late afternoon. This is a pattern that I am sure would benefit most of us. How many overweight chimps have you seen lately? I found it interesting that I had without thinking fallen into a similar pattern, eating fruits for breakfast and having most of my greens in a salad as part of dinner.

Once Victoria understood the importance of getting more greens into her diet, the problem became how to do it. Just chewing them would be a lot of work. Besides the fact that they require being ground into a creamy consistency to become absorbable by the body, many people have low levels of hydrochloric acid in their stomachs. Nutrients cannot be assimilated without both thorough chewing and a stomach pH level of between 1 and 2. Years of eating processed foods make this pH level unlikely. Also, as we age our bodies produce less hydrochloric acid.

Instead of trying to eat large quantities of greens Victoria experimented with "chewing" them in a blender. Initial results were disastrous. The smell and taste were just too nasty. However, she tried adding some bananas to the mixture and the fruit changed everything. Her first green smoothies consisted of one bunch of kale, four bananas, and a quart of water. She and her family loved them.

The result was impressive. They all began to see a difference. Boutenko claims that wrinkles disappeared, her nails became stronger, her vision improved, her energy increased and she felt lighter than she had in years. For weeks Victoria lived on nothing but green smoothies. She stopped craving fatty foods and salt. In the end she lost all cravings for unhealthy foods.

That was my introduction to raw foods. As you can see, it was not about giving up anything that I was eating. I simply added the green smoothie to my diet. For me this was easy. For years I ate only fruit for breakfast, knowing that it is best to eat fruit on an empty stomach, otherwise it tends to ferment behind other slow moving food.

Several years ago I bought a Vita-Mixer blender. This high-powered machine is an essential kitchen appliance for the health conscious human. I knew that blending ruptures plant cells at the microscopic level, making them more available for digestion and more absorbable. I soon was making fruit smoothies every day for breakfast. Now all I had to do was adjust the fruit a little and add greens.

My original green smoothies were simple: two cups of water, four bananas, a handful of kale, and maybe some frozen blueberries or whatever else was in the house. I could never taste the kale. Spinach and romaine lettuce are pretty tasteless, too. Other lettuce may change the fruity flavor so I mostly stuck to the kale, romaine, and spinach.

Now, here is the good part. While not trying hard to give up eating meats and fish, I slowly began to lose interest in them. It wasn't that I didn't want to eat hamburgers anymore; it was simply that they were less attractive by about a half. I didn't want fried food as much either. At this point I was by no means a raw food person or advocate. I just began to feel a little better and the whole experience made me more interested in seeing what other improvements I could make to my diet without causing myself any pain or giving up favorite foods.

I strongly suggest that if you are considering raw foods or any healthy change in your diet, that your first step be that of having one green smoothie a day. Ideally that would be for breakfast, if possible, but it could be later in the day; just try to drink it on an empty stomach because of the fruit. It's painless, it tastes great, and you will feel better by just making that one change.

Additional Reading:

Green For Life. Victoria Boutenko. 2005. Raw Family Publishing.

Chapter 4

Climate Change and Diet

"Livestock are one of the most significant contributors to today's most serious environmental problems. Urgent action is required to remedy the situation."

—HENNING STEINFELD, SENIOR UN FAO OFFICIAL

Did you know that, according to a United Nations report issued in 2006, cattle produce more global warming greenhouse gases than all the cars, trucks, airplanes, buses, and trains combined? Did you know that livestock now use up more than 30 percent of the planet's entire land surface? And I bet you didn't know that producing animal products is damaging the environment through land erosion by overgrazing, depletion of scarce fresh water sources, water pollution, and deforestation (South American rainforest in exchange for American hamburgers).

Methane is 50 times more damaging to the environment than carbon dioxide. Cows, all 1.3 billion of them on the planet, produce more than 100 million tons of the stuff every year. This is the equivalent of 5 billion tons of CO2. Cows, being the ruminants that they are, break down their food by fermenting it. Every time a cow burps and farts, there you go, methane.

Eating animals contributes significantly to global warming. Eating animals contributes to the deforestation of our planet. Eating animals contributes to the destruction of farmland that could be used for feeding human beings. And eating animals contributes to the pollution of our waters. Isn' this a good reason to at least consider changing your diet?

The average person who consumes meats and dairy products requires 20 times the acreage of that of a vegan. The average non-vegan requires 100 times the amount of fresh water to raise the livestock that they will eat. Eating animals has become more than an ethical choice regarding cruelty to other sentient beings, it's about destroying the planet that we live on.

If all of this were not enough, consider that two-thirds of all antibiotics in the United States are given to animals. This is necessary just to keep them alive long enough to get to the slaughterhouse after we have confined them for so long in our factory farms. The overuse of antibiotics is generating a new class of superbugs that are becoming resistant to antibiotics. What happens when antibiotics are no longer of any use?

If we in America stopped eating meat, we would save enough food to feed the 60 million people who starve to death each year on this planet—ten times over! Granted, there are political problems to be overcome, but this gives you an idea of the amount of food we are wasting.

Chapter 5

Victoria Boutenko
and 12 Steps to Raw Foods

"...I did not fully understand the addictive power of cooked foods."

–Gabriel Cousens, M.D.

I enjoyed the simplicity and inspiration of Boutenko's first book so much that I decided to give her raw food book a try. Not that I was intending to become a raw food person, but I was interested in improving my eating habits. One doesn't have to give up cooked foods entirely to benefit from including more raw foods in their diet.

The subtitle of her book is *How to End Your Dependency on Cooked Food.* It is kind of like a 12-step program for food abusers. And most of us, whether we know it or not, do eat food the way addicts consume drugs and alcohol. If you don't believe me, try giving up cooked foods cold turkey for a day and see how fast you start craving your favorite cooked foods, any cooked foods.

I think I was in a good place to begin considering incorporating more raw foods into my life. I knew I needed to lose some weight. I knew from going to my doctor for a physical that my cholesterol was high. And I wanted more energy in my life. Besides, I had seen what it was doing for my daughter and son-in-law.

Part one of Boutenko's book is about how cooking food destroys nutrients and increases the risk for heart disease, diabetes, and cancer. She explains how cooking creates *advanced glycoxidation end products* (AGEs), very toxic molecules that get absorbed by the body and do such nasty things as stiffen muscles (including the heart), reduce flexibility in tendons and ligaments, cause inflammation, and speed up the aging process.

In part two of her book Victoria discusses how we have become addicted to food. We have become dependent on processed cereals and breads, pasteurized drinks, grilled meats and fish. I was amazed at how little I was eating was a living food anymore. Salad and fruit and that's about it for most of us, and those are only side dishes in our diets. Our main meals are almost always cooked foods.

These days I have to laugh to myself when I hear someone describe to me their healthy diets. They'll say "I have hot oatmeal for breakfast with berries on top. Then I have a chicken salad for lunch and fish with rice for dinner." Or something like that. I say to myself, don't they understand that the oatmeal is cooked to a mush, the chicken is filled with antibiotics, and the fish is most likely farmed and they have antibiotics (along with other things), too? Of course, the rice is cooked to death. All this protein is dangerous. What makes all of this even more frustrating is that the so-called nutrition experts on television reinforce this fake healthy diet idea.

The realization that eating cooked food is an addiction is a major contribution to understanding how to improve our dietary habits. No one would think that the typical diet is an addiction, but try to go one day without cooked foods and you will see what I mean. This is a very important point that should not be missed. Cooked foods are an addiction, just as powerful cigarettes, alcohol, drugs, and relationships can be. Knowing this will help you to make healthier food choices.

When I began adding raw foods to my diet it was not the raw food that caused me problems. The more recipes I tried, the more fun I had. My smoothies were delicious. My salads and the interesting dressings that my daughter gave me were totally satisfying. And the mock tuna salad, the flaxseed crackers, and cauliflower "mash potatoes" tasted wonderful. But even with all of these foods, and not being hungry at all, I still wanted to have something cooked at the end of the day, even if it was only a piece of toast and butter. I also craved snacks in the evening, the processed fatty, salty kind.

Victoria does argue that just like an alcoholic we should give up cooked foods entirely, doing so is actually easier in the long run. And I think for some people that would be the way to go. I cannot do this. I don't think I could bring myself to the point where I would never ever want a hamburger again. I may not eat one, but for me knowing that if I really want cooked food I can have it without feeling guilty is important to my sense of freedom. After all, I am trying to be reasonably, rationally, and realistically raw, not absolutely raw.

You may be thinking at this point that the analogy that food is addictive is helpful, but a little of an exaggeration. Well, Victoria points out in her book that plenty of research shows that cooked foods contain opioid peptides that reach the opiate receptors in our nervous systems. These opioid peptides are particularly present in dairy products, meats, poultry, and fish. (Another reason to eat a vegan diet.) Believe it or not, cooked foods are at least somewhat physically addictive.

12 Steps to Raw Foods

Here are Boutenko's 12 steps to transitioning to a raw food diet. I have altered them a little, adding some of my own observations and trying to be brief. I recommend reading the book itself.

1. Become aware that you do have an addiction to cooked foods. Be honest. Can you get through a day without cooked foods and not feel those cravings? Try it.

2. Add healthy foods to your diet; don't think about giving anything up and depriving yourself. Many of our food cravings develop because we do not get enough nutrients. Add a green smoothie and a large salad to your daily diet. Greens are the most nutritious foods on the planet.

3. Learn how to prepare raw food recipes. Get some raw cookbooks. Ask around for good ideas on what to eat. Find out what other people do. Get the tools for making raw foods. Buy a good blender and dehydrator. You probably already have a food processor.

4. Don't judge yourself or others for not eating raw foods. Take the

pressure off yourself, family, and friends. Have fun. Think of this as adding something to your life, not taking anything away. Be reasonable.

5. Avoid temptations. For me this means not keeping cooked foods in the house and not going out to eat very often. I can't help it; if it is in the house I will most likely eat it, so if I don't want cooked foods I don't buy them. It's the same with restaurants. You can only order salad so many times a week. I also find that I am a lot less tempted on a stomach full of my green smoothie. If you are going somewhere where you know you will be tempted—eat first. (If you can't be raw, at least be vegan.)

6. Get support. The encouragement and ideas from my daughter Gina have helped me every step of the way. I could not have made the changes to my diet without her support and help. Support also comes from reading books, raw web sites, newsletters, and attending festivals.

7. Gratitude and forgiveness. Be thankful for learning about this healthy way of living. We may slip at times, but at least we are on the path. We know about raw foods; most people are not even aware of what they are doing to their bodies by eating cooked food all the time. Forgiveness is essential, too. It is hard to make the right choices when we hold grievances against other people...and ourselves.

8. Actualize your dreams. Your life is going to change. You are going to feel happier than you have ever felt before. You will have

more energy and need less sleep. Now you can live your dreams. And the best dreams are those that give back to others.

9. Utilize other healthy practices. Exercise is essential. Move your body. Run, walk, do yoga, swim, incorporate some form of exercise into your daily routine. Get some sunshine.

10. Gain clarity. Spend time with yourself just being aware. Meditate, read; learn to live in the present moment.

11. Find your mission in life. True happiness comes from helping others. Discover what you are meant to do. Where is your passion? What is it that truly gets you excited? Almost every person I know who begins eating a raw vegan diet finds a new sense of spirituality in his or her lives. What does this mean for you?

12. Give support to others. When you help others you are helping yourself. Every time you share what you have learned, you learn it all over again, only better. Your life becomes so much richer. We can't live a healthy lifestyle alone.

I met Victoria and her daughter at the Raw Spirit Festival in Arizona in 2007. Victoria gave an inspiring talk on how she discovered the benefits of green smoothies. Her daughter Valya was working on a raw food documentary, and we talked about how different people experienced healing from various illnesses. I also attended a food preparation demonstration given by Victoria's son Sergei. The children are adults now and were looking quite healthy.

I learned from Victoria Boutenko early on in my raw food journey the importance of adding healthy raw foods to my diet and not to think of this as giving up foods that I loved. I would not have taken the first step had someone told me that I had to give up cooked foods all together. But I could make a green smoothie, and by experimenting they became so enjoyable I had to keep myself from drinking them too fast.

By eating more green leafy vegetables my body became more nourished and being more nourished desired less and less of the junk food and animal foods that I was used to eating. Slowly my tastes we changing. A raw food diet didn't sound quite so strange.

Additional Reading:

12 Steps to Raw Foods: How to End Your Dependency on Cooked Food. Victoria Boutenko. 2007. North Atlantic Books.

Chapter 6

Carnivores, Omnivores, and Herbivores

"Just because we can digest animals, that does not mean we're supposed to, or that it will be good for us. We can digest cardboard."

—MICHAEL BLUEJAY, WRITER AND PUBLISHER

What foods should we eat? How can we know the truth about which foods are healthiest for us? To whom do we listen to when there are so many contradictory voices? Scientists? Nutritionists? Advertisers? Who can we trust?

Ultimately, we have to trust ourselves. We cannot rely on anyone else to give us the answers, because other people and their corporations have their own motivations and agenda. We must think for ourselves. Finding answers always begins with good questions. Here is a good question to ask regarding which foods might make us healthy—for what kind of foods is my body designed?

"We are meat eaters, why else do we have canine teeth." I've heard that said often enough. And, "We are omnivores because we can eat all kinds of foods." That is the most common perception about human beings, that we are omnivores. That is what I believed until I began my research into how the human body is designed.

Natural Carnivores

Carnivores have certain characteristics. They have four feet and tails and claws. They have rough tongues. Canine teeth, *true* canine teeth, are made up of sharp pointy molars and fangs. The jaws of a carnivore have no lateral movement. Carnivores have multiple teats. They sleep between 18 and 20 hours a day. They perspire through their tongues. Carnivores don't drink water; they lap it up with their tongues.

The intestines of carnivores are short and smooth; this is so that flesh does not rot inside them. They also have a high tolerance for microbes in their intestines. The urine and saliva of carnivores is acidic. They have a high tolerance for fat. Carnivores have proportionally large livers, problems digesting sugars, and acid pH levels in their stomachs more than ten times that of humans.

In nature, carnivores prey on other animals, as opposed to grazing on plants. Their diet consists mainly of meat. A true carnivore (or "obligate") must eat meat to live. Guess where they get their vitamins and minerals if they don't eat plants? Two places—the intestines of the animals that they eat is one. The other is the herbivore dung that they also eat! Do either of those sources appeal to you? Thankfully there are other ways to get your nutrients.

Natural Omnivores

Omnivores share many design features of carnivores. They are capable of running down their prey and eating it raw with their bare hands. They have claws and talons. They do not chew their food but tear it into chunks and swallow it whole.

Omnivores are designed to eat both plants and animals. But unlike herbivores, they cannot digest many of the substances in grains or plants that do not produce fruit. Bears are a good example of an omnivore. As far as physical capabilities, omnivores are quite similar to carnivores.

Natural Herbivores

Herbivores are animals adapted to eat plants. The diet of an herbivore is known to vary depending on the season and availability of food. A subgroup within herbivores is frugivores, which mostly eat fruit. (Primates are frugivores.)

Herbivores, not including frugivores and horses, have a four-compartment digestive system, which is needed to digest green leaves and vegetation. Herbivores have intestinal bacteria that aid in digestion. And, differing from carnivores they have no incisors on their upper jaws.

Frugivores

Primates (apes, chimps, man) do not really fit comfortably into any of the above categories. They are not adapted to eating significant amounts of animal or plant matter. Their digestive systems are not designed for meat or grass. But fruit is another thing altogether. It is easily digested and supplies easily assimilated protein, vitamins, and minerals. All frugivores supplement their diets with foliage. (David J. Chivers, Symposium on Nutrition of Non-Ruminant Herbivores, 1988) Humans would be more properly categorized as frugivores rather than as omnivores or herbivores.

The Early Humans

There is no question that early human beings ate other animals. Design or not, microwear on the teeth of specimens show that humans consumed meat. But, there is a question that should be asked—why? Was it out of natural need or was there something else going on? If we look more closely we find that once humans left the tropics and moved into less hospitable lands, they needed alternative sources of nourishment. Seasonal variations in the food supply most likely forced our ancestors to add meat to their diets.

Prior to the changing global climate and change of address, hominids ate diets consisting of plant matter, leaves and fruits. Somewhere between 1 and 2 million B.C. the first true humans appeared and so did some kind of meat eating. It is not known whether they killed their prey or scavenged for it.

In his book *The Rise and Fall of the Third Chimpanzee,* Jared Diamond tells of his "hunting" trip with a tribe in New Guinea that hunts with Stone Age weapons. Apparently, while the men boast of killing large animals, this is rarely the case. (Is this not typical of us men?) The day's hunt resulted in killing two baby birds, several frogs, and a whole lot of mushrooms.

The stone tools used in the hunt were far more advanced than tools found in prehistoric sites, which leads us to believe that back in the day hunters could not have been much more successful. Basically, hunting more likely meant finding carrion (road kill).

While we know that humans ate other animals out of necessity, probably after watching other animals doing it, the human body evolved over millions of years to eat primarily fruits and tender green leaves.

The Omnivores Dilemma?

So what is all this talk about humans being omnivores? It's simple, we have confused the verb "to be able to" with the verb "to be." Just because we *can* eat animals doesn't mean that we *are* animal eaters. I *say* a lot of stupid things, that doesn't mean I *am* a stupid person.

There is no omnivores dilemma, unless you are a grizzly bear, and even then you eat what is available. No, human beings have a body designed for mostly eating fruits with greens thrown in for vitamins and minerals.

Chapter 7

Ann Wigmore and the Hippocrates Health Program

"Let food be your medicine and let medicine be your food."

—HIPPOCRATES OF COS

At midlife in the 1950's Ann Wigmore was a mess. Suffering from gangrene in her legs after a car accident and colon cancer as well, she needed help. Doctors wanted to amputate her legs. She wanted an alternative. Born in Lithuania, and raised partly by her grandmother, she remembered how her grandmother treated wounded soldiers returning from World War I with herbs and weeds.

Ann experimented with various grasses and live foods and eventually healed herself of both the gangrene and the cancer. Not satisfied with overcoming her illnesses, she began research into improving her health. This led her to creating the Hippocrates Health Institute with the help of Viktoras Kulvinskas in Boston in 1958.

Guided by the saying of Hippocrates, "Let food be your medicine," Ann went to work using living foods such as sprouts, juices made from weeds and grass, and fermentation. Wheatgrass became the major element because it was the easiest and cheapest to grow.

Wigmore died in a fire at her institute at the age of 83. Her work continues through institutes such as the Ann Wigmore National Health Institute in Puerto Rico, the Ann Wigmore Foundation in New Mexico, and the Hippocrates Health Institute, which she founded and is currently under the direction of Brian Clement in West Palm Beach, Florida.

The Hippocrates Health Program

The Hippocrates approach has developed over the years but has primarily remained faithful to Wigmore's original research. Enzymes found in living foods are the cornerstone of a healthful diet. Since enzymes are destroyed when food is heated to over 117 degrees, raw uncooked foods are essential.

Vegetables play a key role also, more so than fruits in this program. Young vegetables such as baby greens and sprouts are highly recommended. Sprouts are grown from beans, grains, and seeds. The sprouts are used in salads and juices. To get the most out of fruits and vegetables without stressing the digestive system, juicing is often utilized, especially when fasting.

The juice most associated with Ann Wigmore is wheatgrass juice. Chlorophyll, which is considered the blood of the plant and has characteristics of human blood, can be acquired in concentrated quantities through juicing various grasses; grass grown from wheatberries being the best.

Fermented foods were part of the Hippocrates program under

Wigmore's direction, although they have fallen out of favor recently. Rejuvelac, a fermented drink made of wheatberry, is still widely consumed.

Besides this selection of foods, the Hippocrates program includes ideas regarding the proper combining of foods in a meal and cleansing. Eating certain foods together can cause digestion problems and nutrients not to be absorbed properly. Cleansing is needed to rid the body of toxins acquired through years of eating the standard American diet.

Enzymes

Probably the best reason for wanting to eat raw foods is the enzymes. Cooking food kills the enzymes in the food. According to the Hippocrates theory, people are given only a certain amount of enzymes at birth. We lose enzymes when our bodies fight illness, disease, and stress. A deficiency in enzymes brings about many kinds of health issues such as heart disease and certain cancers.

By eating raw foods we are able to replenish enzymes and rebuild our bodies. Wigmore called enzymes the body's labor force. Enzymes are the life energy that is metabolism at work. The faster one uses up one's enzyme supply, the faster one dies.

Wigmore wrote that enzymes were the key to the Hippocrates Diet. By predigesting and breaking down foods in the stomach, nutrients are more readily absorbed and utilized by the body. Then the digestive system does not have to work so hard, making more energy available for living and protection from illness.

When a person eats a primarily raw diet, he or she is making it easier on themselves to cleanse, repair, and rebuild their bodies. And enzymes are the reason. By not cooking food you preserve the enzymes, which are needed for good health.

Wheatgrass

When you think of Ann Wigmore, you have to think wheatgrass. Most of us do not know the major role that grass has and still does play in the development of life on this planet. The grain that we make bread from comes from the seeds of grass. And, of course, so many animals survive on grass. Grasses have been used for centuries as medicine in Eastern and Western cultures. Chlorophyll is the key ingredient in grass that makes it so valuable.

Chlorophyll helps to oxygenate blood. Diets high in fat and protein cause blood to be depleted of oxygen. This in turn causes people to have less energy, poor digestion, and weaker immune systems. It may also cause cancer.

Exercise certainly is important to get oxygen into the blood. But foods too can help. Raw fruits, vegetables, juices, and sprouts contain chlorophyll, which is nearly identical to human blood in the sense that it carries oxygen.

Wigmore discovered that one of the best sources of chlorophyll was wheatgrass juice. (Wheatgrass itself is too fibrous to eat.) Agricultural chemist Charles Schnabel did the original research back in the 1930's. He dried the grass and sold it in cans. According to Wigmore's writings, the chlorophyll in wheatgrass is good for cleansing the blood, internal organs, and the digestive system. It also lowers blood pressure by dilating arteries. The red blood cell count is increased, and metabolism is stimulated.

Wheatgrass chlorophyll is concentrated with vitamins, minerals, and living enzymes. Wigmore used it to treat ulcers and colitis, cleanse the colon, and strengthen the immune system. She also used other grasses and seeds to extract chlorophyll from plants.

Brian Clement, the current director of the Hippocrates Institute, writes that wheatgrass chlorophyll cleanses the body of toxins and suppresses bacterial growth. Wheatgrass juice is not very stable and should be consumed shortly after preparation. Also, because it is so strong it may cause nausea or indigestion.

Sprouts

Another key contribution that Ann Wigmore made to a better understanding towards the components of a healthier diet is that sprouts are a source of super nutrition. According to her theory, enzymes reach their peak activity between the second and seventh day after sprouting.

Historically, sprouts have been used in various cultures to heal many illnesses. The Chinese discovered them thousands of years ago. Sprouts contain significant levels of amino acids (the building blocks of protein), high levels of vitamins and minerals, and when included with other foods make them more nutritious.

"Being eaten whilst extremely young, "alive" and rapidly developing, sprouts have been acclaimed as the "most enzyme-rich food on the planet". Estimates suggest there can be up to 100 times more enzymes in sprouts than in fruit and vegetables, depending on the particular type of enzyme and the variety of seed being sprouted. The period of greatest enzyme activity in sprouts is generally between germination and 7 days of age."

—Isabell Shipard, Naturopath

The germination of seeds, grains, nuts, and legumes, is a simple first step in the sprouting process that anyone could easily incorporate into their eating habits. Seeds contain metabolic inhibitors that protect it while in its dormant state. These inhibitors make the seeds less useable by the human body. Soaking, which begins the germination process, removes the inhibitors and the seed begins to grow. At this point starches become sugars, proteins become amino acids, and fats become soluble fatty acids.

I soak various nuts and seeds, and I can tell you that they taste much better after soaking. The only thing is that they turn moldy quicker when traveling if you don't keep them refrigerated.

The best thing about sprouts is that they can be grown at home cheaply and easily. There are even automatic sprouters available making this facet of building a healthy diet quite painless.

Juices

While other people are more famous for promoting the value of drinking fruit and vegetable juices, Wigmore was one of the first to actually include juicing in her diet. Wheatgrass was not the only thing that she extracted juice from.

Besides juicing fruits, vegetables and sprouts make an important contribution to the Hippocrates diet. Sprouts are considered the ultimate living food to juice because they are the most alive of all living foods. Vegetables are added for flavor.

The benefit in juicing is that vitamins, minerals, enzymes, amino acids, and sugars can be consumed without putting a lot of stress on the digestive system. Juicing also adds electrolytes and oxygen to the blood. Juices make the perfect drink to have when fasting. Juicing is one way to supplement your diet without using supplements made in a chemistry lab.

Fruits and Vegetables

The Hippocrates Health Program places a much greater emphasis on vegetables than on fruits. In fact, vegetables make up the largest part of the diet. It is recommended that large salads be eaten. What I mean by large salads is that, according to Wigmore, it should take a half hour to eat!

Besides the obvious benefit of vitamins, minerals, and protein, vegetables provide the natural fiber needed to exercise the colon and remove waste from our systems. Baby greens are probably the best of all vegetables to eat.

Sea vegetables play an important role in the Hippocrates diet. Because they are grown in the ocean, they are able to make minerals and trace elements available to humans which are not available from land-grown plants. Dulse, kelp, nori, wakame, and others should be eaten daily. A couple of tablespoons would be enough. Dulse and kelp can be used to replace salt in your diet.

If you follow the Hippocrates plan you will not be eating a lot of fruit; only two to five pieces a day are recommended. However, Wigmore does recommend fruit, especially bananas, to lose weight. My understanding is that while the emphasis is placed on eating vegetables, significant consumption of fruit isn't discouraged.

Rejuvelac

Grind up half a cup of sprouted wheatberries, put them in a couple of jars full of water, cover with cheesecloth, and let it sit for three or four days and you have Rejuvelac. Ann Wigmore recommended that eight to sixteen ounces of this fermented beverage be consumed every day. Wigmore felt that fermented foods were good for the colon. This, however, has fallen out of favor at the Institute today, although Rejuvelac is still popular among many raw fooders.

Cleansing and Fasting

It often happens that when people begin eating a mostly raw food diet, in the beginning, they go through a cleansing period and feel sick instead of better. This is the cleaning stage. As the body rids itself of toxins many symptoms of illness arise. This is just the discomfort of a lot of accumulated waste leaving your system.

Wigmore recommended watermelon and watermelon juice for breakfast, Rejuvelac or juices between meals, fruit, and two large salads a day, in addition to supplementing the diet with wheatgrass juice, sea vegetables, and green drinks made of sprouts and vegetables. Rest, walking, and stretching, were also included.

Cleansing the colon is a big part of the Hippocrates program. The colon is the primary organ of solid waste disposal for the body. Years of eating foods that shouldn't have been eaten leave it clogged up and in poor shape to extract vital nutrients. In addition, most people have little healthy bacteria and lots of the bad kind due to taking antibiotics by prescription or consumed in the meat that we eat.

Besides eating raw foods, Wigmore was a big fan of enemas, wheatgrass implants, and colonics. In some parts of the raw food movement this has been taken to the extreme and it appears that some people even get addicted to them. I don't know how, but to hear them talk about it, well, let's not go there.

Fasting, while not originally recommended by Wigmore, is part of the Hippocrates program today. A fast of one day a week on juices and purified water is part of the detoxification process. Rather than fast on just water, which will release massive amounts of toxins from their stored places in the body, a fruit and vegetable juice fast slows the process down, making the faster more comfortable and in a less weakened state.

Food Combining

A healthy diet is not only about what you eat, it also involves when you eat it. Most of us eat more than one food at a time. Eating certain foods together, known as food combining, can cause the digestive process to become derailed, and then we will not absorb all the nutrients that we could from what we are eating.

One objective of the Hippocrates diet is to allow foods to be quickly and easily utilized by the body and then eliminated. An understanding of proper food combining will help this to happen. It is not enough to eat living foods; they have to be eaten in a health-promoting combination.

Foods entering the body have to be digested to release their nutrients. Two aspects of digestion are affected by how those foods are combined. One is that protein foods entering the stomach require acidic juices to be digested, while starchy foods need alkaline juices. When both kinds of foods enter the stomach together, they tend to cancel out each other's digestive juices.

The other aspect of digestion is that different foods digest at different rates. If a food that digests at a faster rate comes in after one that digests at a slower rate, the faster food will not digest properly, causing digestion to slow down and poor absorption of nutrients.

Proper food combining includes the following guidelines:

1. Mono meals are the best. This means eating only one food at a sitting. Watermelon for breakfast makes a great cleansing mono meal.

2. All melons, because they are digested so much faster than any other food, should always be eaten alone.

3. Fruits come in three categories: acid, subacid, and sweet. They have different amounts of sugar and water and are digested at different rates. Subacid fruits can be eaten with acidic or sweet, but acidic and sweet should not be eaten together.

4. Don't mix fruits and vegetables.

5. Don't mix starches with proteins.

6. Don't drink with a meal.

7. Eat raw foods before cooked.

Some of this may sound familiar to you if you have ever read *Fit For Life* by Harvey and Marilyn Diamond. The Diamonds popularized the idea of proper food combining back in 1985. Food combining is also a part of the Natural Hygiene approach to raw foods.

The Three Phases

Part of the Hippocrates Health Program today includes the concept that becoming a living-foods vegan is a twenty-one-year journey. It is holistic in the sense that the program involves the body, mind, and spirit.

Phase one answers the question: what am I made of? During the first seven years you rebuild and energize your body. Physical changes include more strength and flexibility, a better digestive system, proper weight, and excellent health.

Phase two concerns the mind and answers the question: who am I? After achieving a more comfortable physical presence, the practitioner works for the next seven years toward better emotional health. Once physical problems have been overcome, a person can then work on the mental aspect. Some, including myself, would argue that the mental should come before or at least at the same time.

The third phase asks the question: Why am I here? This is the spiritual phase, and now that mind and body are healthy, one can begin a spiritual journey. Again, it could be questioned whether it is necessary to wait fourteen years before considering spirituality and health. I believe that Brian Clement developed the concept of the three phases and I am not sure that Ann Wigmore supported the idea.

The Best of Ann Wigmore and the Hippocrates Health Program

Ann Wigmore has to be appreciated for being a pioneer herald of raw foods and living enzymes. I know intuitively that raw is better than cooked, but why? It's the enzymes. Knowing this makes it a little easier to…digest.

Germinate seeds and get greater nutrition from them. It's simple and quick. Grow your own sprouts. Ann Wigmore's focus on the benefits of sprouts is something that most people overlook. It makes sense to germinate and sprout seeds right in our own homes. Sprouts are a living food at its peak.

While I can't say that wheatgrass juice is something everyone should be drinking, I do applaud Wigmore for calling attention to the benefits of chlorophyll. The consumption of green leafy plants cannot be emphasized enough.

Lastly, and possibly most important, is the benefit of drinking vegetable juice. I had been a big juicing fan back in the 1980's thanks to The Juiceman, Jay Kordich, but I stopped juicing a number of years ago. I got tired of drinking five pound bags of carrots every day. But Wigmore explains why we should juice all kinds of vegetables as a healthy supplement to eating them. I also very much like the idea of fasting one day a week on juices to give the digestive system a rest.

Further Reading:

The Hippocrates Diet and Health Program. Ann Wigmore. 1984. Avery. (This book is an excellent introduction to Ann Wigmore's philosophy of health. It also contains instructions for growing sprouts, gardening indoors, and many of her own recipes.)

Living Foods for Optimum Health: Your Complete Guide to the Healing Power of Raw Foods. Brian R. Clement with Theresa Foy DiGeronimo. 1998. Three Rivers Press. (Brian Clement has been the director of the Hippocrates Institute for more than twenty-five years.

Chapter 8

Brainwashed!

"Brainwashing: The application of a concentrated means of persuasion, such as an advertising campaign or repeated suggestion, in order to develop a specific belief or motivation."

−THE AMERICAN HERITAGE DICTIONARY

Brainwashed is a strong, emotionally charged word. But it is appropriate when we consider our beliefs about food. Ever since the 1940's, when Danish scientists discovered a link between the consumption of animal products and disease, there has been a concerted effort on the part of the food industry to brainwash the American people.

The American Meat Institute, the National Dairy Council, the National Dairy Promotion Board, the Cattlemen's Beef Association, among others, spend hundreds of millions of dollars every year with the express purpose of increasing the demand for animal products. They do this in incredibly devious ways.

*"For modern animal agriculture, the less the consumer knows-
about what's happening before the meat hits the plate,
the better…"*

—PETER CHEEKE, PROFESSOR OF ANIMAL SCIENCE

The obvious advertising that we see on television and in newsprint is only the tip of the iceberg. The hideousness of the work being done to convince you and me to eat more animals is executed behind the scenes, in the committees that make up the reports that make advertising more convincing and make the truth about what is healthy to eat and what is not more confusing.

Did you know: In the waiting rooms of nearly all 50,000 family doctor's offices in the United States, sent free, published by the American Academy of Family Physicians, lies a glossy 243 page magazine. It is called *Family Doctor: Your Essential Guide to Health and Well-being.* In one issue, on pages two and three, you will find an ad for McDonald's. Later in the publication, opposite an article on "Pregnancy and Newborn" is an ad touting the benefits of eating tuna fish. Logging into the *Family Doctor's* web site you will find "proud" sponsors such as the Atkins diet people (eat lots of meat and fat), Too Tarts (selling spray candy of all things), Sinfully Delicious (candy without calories), Bimbo (sugary pastries), PepsiCo (selling Lays potato chips, Pepsi, Cheetos and Doritos), 3-A Day (pushing the benefits of three servings a day of milk, cheese, and yogurt) and Wyeth

Pharmaceuticals (selling Advil and the antidepressant Effexor). All of this from the people who claim to be "your essential guide to health and well-being."

Here is one area in how this brainwashing works: An Act of Congress created the National Academy of Sciences (NAS) in 1863. NAS created IOM (Institute of Medicine), which has the role of advising the government on issues of health. A part of the IOM is the Food and Nutrition Board (FNB), which makes recommendations concerning food, nutrition, and health. Since 1940 the FNB has been establishing principles and guidelines for adequate nutrition and the relationship between food and health.

The Food and Nutrition Board publishes highly respected findings telling the American people what is good to eat and what is not. They have been doing this since before many of us were born. We grew up with their published reports informing everything and everyone about nutrition.

Just for fun I googled several of the current members of the board. I started with the board chairman, pediatrician Dr. Dennis M. Bier. This is what I found in his conflict of interest statement for the American Journal of Clinical Nutrition: Dr. Bier consults for ConAgra Foods (they produce many brands of processed foods and meat products), Mars (the candy people), and McDonald's (you know who they are).

The previous chairman was a paid consultant for the National Dairy Council, Nestle, and Dannon. He is now a senior executive for a large food corporation. You might suspect that this is a payoff for his good work on their agenda.

Next down the line, I looked up vice-chair Michael Doyle. According to Integrity in Science, he has received numerous grants from the American Meat Institute and is a paid consultant of Kraft Foods.

Jim Riviere is a paid consultant for numerous drug companies. Fergus Clydesdale receives funding from Kraft and owns stock in several food companies. Six of the eleven members have direct ties to the dairy industry.

While government scientists cannot receive personal compensation from the food industry, these academics serving on the FNB board can. Conflicts of interest abound. And these are the people given the responsibility to "render authoritative judgment on the relationships among food intake, nutrition, and health."

"Although sponsorship by food companies is ubiquitous among academics and practitioners in the fields of nutrition, food, and agriculture, our community has paid scant attention to the conflicts of interest that might arise from this. Like drug and tobacco companies, food companies often sponsor academic work (and in fact many drug and tobacco companies own food companies)."

–MARION NESTLE, DEPT. OF FOOD AND NUTRITION, NYU

It was this committee that in its most recent report made recommendations stating that for good health adults should get 45% to 65% of their calories from carbohydrates, 20% to 35% from fat, and 10% to 35% from protein. They also said that it was okay to consume up to 25% of total calories from added sugars found in soft drinks, candy, pastries, and other sweets. We are told that by following these guidelines we will minimize the risk for chronic disease.

That means that you could have a bowl of Fruit Loops and a Snickers bar for breakfast, a cheeseburger for lunch, and pizza and soda for dinner, and still be within the FNB guidelines. Essentially, they're telling you to eat whatever you want.

"My eight-year-old stepson, upon finding out that I don't eat meat or anything coming from an animal, told me that I will never develop any muscles because muscles come from animals."

–KIRSTEN, INTERNET E-MAIL POSTING

The FNB and committee members affect how people eat in a variety of ways. They establish the Food Pyramid. They influence the National School Lunch and Breakfast programs, the Food Stamp Program, and the Women, Infants and Children Supplemental Feeding Program. Approximately thirty-five million Americans are provided food by government programs based on what the Food and Nutrition Board recommends. In addition, what we eat in hospitals and nursing homes is determined by FNB.

The brainwashing doesn't stop there. The food industry has its hands in many other important avenues of influence. Nutrition journals take money from the food industry and companies through corporate sponsorships. The food companies also sponsor nutrition conferences and the publication of academic papers. Sponsored papers are not even subjected to peer-review.

The Dairy Council and the National Cattleman's Beef Association sponsor research sessions. Travel funds, gifts, and meals are used to gain influence and interest in products being sold.

Associations themselves cooperate. The American Heart Association receives money from Kellogg's, and then gives its seal of approval on foods like Frosted Flakes, Fruity Marshmallow Krispies, and Pop-Tarts. The American Dietetic Association receives significant funding from McDonald's, Kellogg's, and other food companies.

The entire system of official information about food is under the control of the food industry. Is there any wonder why in America cancer, heart disease, diabetes, and obesity have become epidemics? And if that doesn't kill you, the health care system will (the third leading cause of death in the US). We are being brainwashed into eating foods that are killing us, and the food industry profits from our illness. At the same time big medicine is kept in business. They have major incentives to keep their mouths shut; otherwise they would be out of work.

The human mind is an interesting thing. It is capable of believing whatever it wants to. We select what we want to see and hear and believe. We want to believe that the big steak we are about to eat is good for us, providing us with protein. If it isn't the steak, well then, the chicken, or the fish. Hey, pizza is a health food; after all it contains all the food groups.

You will never hear the food experts on the Today Show or Good Morning America tell you the truth about nutrition. Why? Because if they did, their sponsors would stop advertising with them. Even here the food industry manipulates the truth. The only place we find real research answers is where there is no influence from money—books and unsponsored Internet sites.

It is my hope that after reading this you will open your mind to some new possibilities. Just being aware of how you have been lied to and used all of these years will free you from much of the misinformation that you have been fed. Now we will get to ideas that are not being forced upon you so that someone, somewhere can make a buck. Let's get at the raw truth.

Chapter 9

David Wolfe, Superfoods, and the Best Day Ever

"Life is generous to those who pursue their destiny."

—DAVID WOLFE

David Wolfe may very well be the most important figure in the raw food movement. He is the rock star (drummer in the Healing Waters Band), the super food king (Sunfood Nutrition), and the creator of the Sunfood Diet Success System. David Wolfe is raw foods on steroids. You have to like a guy who has made chocolate into a health food and always celebrates the best day ever.

For all the hype (he claims to be the world's leading voice on raw nutrition), the groupies (Goji Girl, etc.), the nickname (Avocado), the unusual hairstyle, the relentless promotion of products (the world's largest distributor of anything to do with raw food), Wolfe is probably the best overall resource and inspiration when it comes to raw foods. His book *The Sunfood Diet Success System* is one of the most comprehensive books on raw food available. He not only covers most aspects of becoming a raw foodist, but he offers plenty of motivational material besides.

Wolfe gives nearly a hundred lectures a year along with raw adventure retreats throughout the world. His goal, in his own words, is *"to become the greatest promoter of The Raw Food Diet in the history of the world."* He maintains at least three different web sites to do this. To his credit he seems to draw from many different raw food authorities and teachers.

While not being a Natural Hygienist, his diet tends to conform closely to its precepts. According to Wolfe in an interview on the *Living and Raw Foods* website, his diet is made up of 80 percent fruit, 15 percent vegetables, and 5 percent nuts. He promotes a modified fruitarian diet and the more wild food, the better. He also believes in just going raw cold turkey. Wolfe quotes Stephen Arlin, "You crave whatever is in your bloodstream." Better to get cooked food out sooner rather than later. This is easier than becoming raw slowly.

Chocolate

You cannot talk about David Wolfe without first talking about chocolate, or what the Aztecs called *cachooatl* and the Spaniards called cacao. Cacao is the bean that chocolate is made from. But it isn't chocolate itself that raw foodists are interested in; it is the cacao bean and its amazing health properties.

The cacao nut was so important in ancient Central America that it was used as money. Workers were paid in cacao. Cacao was used as standard currency in Mexico until 1887.

Magnesium is the main reason for eating cacao. According to Wolfe magnesium is the most deficient dietary mineral in America.

Cacao is the major source of magnesium in nature. Magnesium is necessary for strong heart muscle, a healthy brain, muscle relaxation, bone formation, and good bowel movements.

The cacao bean is one of the best sources of antioxidants, far superior to blueberries. It also contains tryptophan in large quantities. Tryptophan is necessary for the body to produce serotonin, which is a wonderful mood enhancer. Wolfe calls cacao nature's Prozac.

Superfoods

Cacao is a superfood, but not the only one that Wolfe considers important to human health. Others include fresh water algae (spirulina and blue-green algae), sea vegetables (kelp), maca, goji berries, aloe vera, bee products, hemp seed, and Incan berries.

Superfoods are special because they contain high concentrations of vitamins, minerals, trace minerals, enzymes, and proteins. According to Wolfe, they make it easier to detoxify, maintain ideal weight, and transition to a raw food diet. They eliminate the need for food supplements. In a sense, they *are* food supplements.

Fresh water algae (Spirulina and Blue-Green Algae from Klamath Lake) is a concentrated source of chlorophyll, protein, antioxidants, and omega 3 fatty acids. Algae may be the most nutrient dense food in the world. The soft cell walls make it easily absorbed and utilized by the body. Algae is also a source of B12. In one form or another, algae should be a daily addition to every diet.

Sea vegetables are basically seaweeds. They are neither plant nor animal and are another form of algae. Some sea vegetables are kelp, dulse, sea lettuce, nori, and wakame. Sea Vegetables are the foundation of the food chain and probably led to the formation of the first invertebrates.

The essential elements and trace minerals found in sea vegetables are important to our endocrine system and the regulation of the body's metabolism. Sea vegetables help cleanse the intestinal tract and lymph system, stabilize blood sugar levels, purify and alkalize the blood, and inhibit cancer cell growth. They also promote healthy thyroid functioning, reduce cardiovascular problems, and have been shown to be anti-inflammatory. Powdered sea vegetables can be used to replace table salt and are excellent sprinkled on salads.

Maca is a superfood that is found high in the Andes of Peru. It is a root vegetable and considered to have medicinal qualities. Maca is similar to a radish or turnip. Consumption of the maca root powder is shown to strengthen the immune system, increase energy, endurance and libido. In tests mice have shown that it reduces enlarged prostates.

The major benefits of maca are reduced risk of prostate cancer, increased stamina, improved memory, stress relief, and help in overcoming depression. Maca is touted as an alternative to Viagra. It also improves fertility.

Goji berries, known as wolfberry in America, are touted by David Wolfe as possibly the most nutritionally dense food on the planet. (I think he says this about a lot of fruits and vegetables.) In the Chinese system of herbal medicine, Goji berries rank number one out of more than eight thousand. They have been used for healing for over two thousand years.

The goji berry is a complete source of protein, containing all eight essential amino acids. Goji berries have twice the amount of antioxidants as blueberries. According to Wolfe, goji berries are the only food known to stimulate the human growth hormone. This makes the berry "the world's greatest anti-aging superfood."

The Food Triangle

David Wolfe teaches that the secret to succeeding on a raw food diet and achieving high levels of health is a balance between three essential classes of foods. Those classes make up the raw food triangle. Through his experiences of meeting hundreds of raw foodists and studying what works and what doesn't, he discovered a pattern.

The three essential foods are green-leafy vegetables, sweet fruits, and fatty foods. The three provide chlorophyll, sugars, and fats. Lacking any of these foods results in nutritional imbalance. In Wolfe's travels, all successful raw foodists followed this pattern. People lacking one of these food groups always ran into trouble.

In most cases Wolfe calls for the three foods to be eaten in equal quantities. And for the best results, all three food classes should be eaten every day. David personally suggests having sweet fruits as the main meal in the morning, green-leafy vegetables at lunch, and fats in the evening.

Green-leafy vegetables provide chlorophyll; chlorophyll is the "blood" of plants. Just like in the old Popeye cartoons, we get our strength from spinach (and other greens). They provide us with calcium, iron, magnesium, and other minerals. Greens help detoxify the liver. They alkalize our body chemistry, balancing acid-forming minerals found in nuts, seeds, avocados, and animal products.

Sugar comes to us through sweet fruits. Sugar is the fuel that runs our bodies and brains. We need fruit for energy. However, too much fruit can overstimulate the endocrine system and acidify the blood. Therefore, fruit needs to be balanced with green-leafy vegetables and fats. (This is something the natural hygiene people would disagree with.)

Wolfe warns us to avoid refined sugar, which should not come as a surprise, but he also points out that hybrid fruits (seedless) should be avoided. Seedless bananas, watermelon, grapes, oranges, etc. contain sugar that can act like processed sugar. A diet high in these fruits can lead to constipation, dehydration, and a slightly diabetic situation. This is avoided with lots of dark green-leafy vegetables and exercise.

Natural raw fats are the third part of Wolfe's health equation. Raw plant foods such as avocados, durians, young coconuts, nuts, seeds, and oils provide essential fatty acids needed to lubricate mucus linings and the body joints. They also are critical for skin and hair beauty. These plant foods also contain omega 6 and omega 3 fatty acids.

One benefit of having fat with fruits, or fatty fruits like avocado, is that the fat slows the release of sugar into the digestive track. This makes for a longer release time and more energy over a longer time.

Plant fats contain no cholesterol. Raw plant fats help the body access and absorb the minerals in green-leafy vegetables. They will not cause excess weight gain as cooked fats do. Plant fats insulate the nerves and counteract against environmental pollution.

Here is something that those of us new to the raw vegan diet need to understand: when you are feeling hungry and feel the need for heavy protein food, that is not what your body is asking for. At times like these it is not protein that your body wants, it's fat. Wolfe states that plant fats are an excellent bridge from cooked foods to a raw food diet. And if you are going to be eating nuts and seeds, it is best to soak them first. This removes their enzyme inhibitors, their coverings that prevent them from sprouting.

Superfood Smoothie

The cornerstone to David Wolfe's raw food diet, in his own personal life, is a superfood smoothie. In a number of videos and interviews he discusses his daily smoothie and how he makes it.

The following recipe is taken from an interview demonstration Wolfe gave on the Internet television show *Healthy Living* shown on Supreme Master Television. The smoothie begins with a base of coconut water taken from a young Thai coconut. As an alternative you could use spring water, tea, or even coffee. Along with the water of the coconut Wolfe adds the meat to the drink also.

Next comes cacao. Wolfe uses about a tablespoon of the cacao nibs, a half tablespoon of the powder, and a half-tablespoon of the cacao butter.

Following the base of water and cacao Wolfe includes two cups of frozen berries—strawberries, raspberries and/or wild blueberries. He suggests that including foods of the full spectrum of color is best because that provides all of the possible antioxidants. In addition to the frozen fruit, acai and goji berries are used.

Wolfe then puts in a handful of cashews for fat and flavor along with superfoods maca, hemp seeds, and spirulina. And that is it—David Wolfe's superfood smoothie. David usually has this as a late morning breakfast. He has a large salad at 7 pm for his other meal of the day and snacks on fruits, nuts and seeds, and juices in between.

The Best of David Wolfe

Chocolate. Superfoods. Passion. Chocolate added to a superfood smoothie is heaven. When I began adding raw cacao powder to my afternoon smoothies I simply began looking forward to them as if I were having a real milk shake treat, not a substitute. While I don't want to overdo it with cacao, the addition of cacao to my smoothies and the raw ice cream that I make with durian (another fruit introduced to me by Wolfe) has made eating raw foods so much more enjoyable.

The addition of superfoods to my smoothies is another part of my diet that David Wolfe has changed. In the past I took supplements in the form of pills. Now I take them in the form of superfoods. A little spirulina, maca, and dulse in addition to lots of green-leafy vegetables and I feel that I cover all my bases.

Finally, I can't talk about David Wolfe without talking about passion for raw food. Listening to him or watching him is inspiring to the point of making one get up and doing something. If raw food can make David so energetic, why can't it do the same for me? I've sat through one of his four-hour lectures and he just does not want to stop. He is doing something right.

Additional Reading:

Naked Chocolate. David Wolfe and Shazzie. 2005. Maul Brothers Publishing.

The Sunfood Diet Success System. David Wolfe. 2006. Maul Brothers Publishing.

Chapter 10

The Ethical Considerations
of Eating Animals

"If man's aspirations towards right living are serious... he will first abstain from animal food because... its use is simply immoral, as it requires the performance of an act which is contrary to moral feeling - killing."

–LEO TOLSTOY

On June 11, 1963 in downtown Saigon, a Buddhist monk, Thich Quang Duc, burned himself to death protesting the persecution of Buddhists by the South Vietnamese government. Was the monk's suicide an immoral act?

An ethical discussion is not about the absolute rightness or wrongness of an action, because each act's judgment is determined by the intention of the person and the content of the situation.

When Thich Quang Duc killed himself, he was sacrificing his life for a greater cause. Another person may be in so much pain that they cannot stand to live for another day and therefore decide to commit suicide. Yet another may do it accidentally with a drug overdose. And still another may have a well thought out plan to just end their life.

All with different intentions, all with different contexts. Ethical actions are evaluated not as black and white, but within a spectrum of colors.

When we consider the ethics of eating animals, a number of considerations and circumstances must be taken into account.

For a moment, let's think about the first time a human being took a bite of an animal. We know that primates evolved eating mostly fruits, a modest amount of leaves, and an occasional insect or two along with bark and other plant matter. What was it like to go from this to eating that very first carcass?

A question more appropriate to our discussion would be—why eat an animal in the first place? The answer probably wasn't because of being in the mood for a nice prime rib. They were probably starving and had seen other animals doing it. They probably didn't have a choice, they did it to survive. As the human population increased and moved out into less hospitable lands, eventually they needed another source of food. And since humans *could* eat meat, they did.

Over time a way to make fire was discovered and cooking animals must have made the experience much more palatable. Ethically speaking, no one could fault eating animals under these circumstances. Human beings became meateaters.

Fast-forward to today and wealthy societies eat more animals than ever, even though we don't need to. In America, in 2000, the average American ate 195 pounds of red meat, poultry and fish.

When there are alternatives to eating other animals, as there are now in America, then we have to ask the question if this is ethical.

Again, there is no black or white answer. Some people just don't think about it, they have never even considered if it was wrong to eat hamburgers or Chicken McNuggets. There is no intention there to do wrong. Other people have thought about it and decided that there is nothing wrong with killing other animals to eat them. End of story.

And if the killing of animals because we enjoy the taste of meat is accepted, I'd like to make the stories that we tell ourselves so that we will not feel guilt about it a little more complicated. Instead of an all-or-nothing decision, why not look at our choice to eat animals as one of good, better, and best. My ex-wife's great aunt Zia used to ask me if I liked to drink wine. She would say, "If-a-you drink wine, that's-a-good. If-a-you don't, that's-a-better."

Maybe eating animals isn't the worst thing in the world to do. Certainly it's not a crime. But maybe there are better ways of eating. Is it better to eat 100 pounds of animals a year than 195? Is it better to eat 100 pounds of shrimp than of veal? The philosopher Ken Wilber says that it is better to eat a carrot than a cow. Why? Why is it better to eat a carrot than a cow?

It's better to eat a carrot than a cow because there is less suffering involved. It's better to eat a scallop than a chicken because there is less suffering. If you are getting your animals the old-fashioned way, hunting, you could argue this point, but if your food is coming from the supermarket…

The purpose of this chapter is not to tell you what is right and wrong. You must decide that. Our purpose here is just to consider the possibility that eating animals may be an unconscious conflict with our moral precepts, which brings us unwanted consequences. The health of the body is not only about the physical components; there is a mental and spiritual side of the human experience. How we think and behave ethically most assuredly shows up in our bodies.

"The greatness of a nation and its moral progress can be judged by the way its animals are treated."

–MAHATMA GANDHI

Why is it that dogs get Christmas presents and pigs get to be Christmas ham?

Factory Farming

The earliest humans picked their food from trees. Living in the topics, they comfortably ate wild fruit, leafy greens, some nuts, seeds, and a few insects. As the population grew, this paradise could not support so many people, and we began to expand into less hospitable territory.

It was at this time that we began eating other types of food. We had no other choice. However, by then our digestive systems were already formed. We were, and still are, naturally frugivores.

To survive, we began eating wild animals, then we learned to cultivate grains (the seeds of grasses). And most recently, we learned to cultivate animals as well. Under pressure not just to feed a population but to also make a profit, humankind developed what is now called factory farming.

Cows

Since the 1980's the beef industry has been run by four huge corporations. Since there is no federal law governing the welfare of farm animals, cruelty is perfectly acceptable, as long as you are a farmer. This opens the door to the hideousness of factory farming.

After spending the first six months of life on the range feeding on their natural food—grass, cattle are shipped to feedlots where they will spend the rest of their lives eating unnatural food solely for the purposes of marbleizing their flesh with fat. Instead of grass, cattle in feedlots are fed corn. (Their feed also contains chicken and pig meat, beef blood and fat, along with chicken litter, which contains fecal matter. The average cow gets to eat over sixty pounds of this chicken litter.)

Why are cows fed corn? Economics. Corn, with its government subsidies, is dirt-cheap. The only problem with this is that since cows are not designed to eat corn, they must be kept alive by injecting them with antibiotics. (They are also pumped up with synthetic growth hormones.)

Stuffed into crowded feedlots, the cattle sleep in their own shit, they breathe in air thick with bacteria and particulate matter, and need more medication to fight respiratory disease. By the time they go in for slaughter, the manure is caked into their hides. Is it any wonder that microbes like E. Coli are found in beef? Now they are irradiating the meat to kill the microbes. I wonder which is worse.

We won't get into the slaughtering process, which is so bad that they will not let anyone in to see what they are doing. Beef, may be "real food for real people," but it's a really miserable life if you happen to be one. If you would like to see what does go on in the slaughterhouse, watch the youtube video entitled *"Earthlings."*

Pigs

Pigs do not have it any better than cows. Factory farmed pigs (ninety percent of all pork comes to us from these meat factories) spend their entire lives inside, contained in steel pens. No straw, nothing to do all day long. They stand or lie on concrete floors. Sows are kept in stalls so small they cannot even turn around. These are intelligent, sensitive, and social animals. Next time you order baby back ribs or bring home the bacon, consider the suffering of these animals.

Chickens

Ninety-five percent of all chickens are raised under factory farm conditions. They are kept in cages and allowed to live in a space the size of an eight by eleven-inch piece of paper. They cannot move, they cannot get away from more aggressive animals. They have nervous systems similar to ours.

The ammonia levels in the buildings cause respiratory disease. They are in constant pain because they are bred for fast growth. They become so big their bones cannot support their own weight. Like cows, they stand in their own shit all day long. High intensity farming like this is a breeding ground for illnesses like the avian flu. The birds are pumped with antibiotics to keep them alive.

The sensitive beak, full of nerve endings, is seared off with a hot blade to prevent fighting and pecking. When it comes time to die, many of them are scalded alive. Unskilled, low-paid workers soon become desensitized and treat them terribly.

Dairy Cows

Do you think that dairy cows live the idyllic lives depicted on milk cartons? Think again. They are not allowed to graze on grass, but are kept indoors. When kept outside, they live in dirt lots. They are bred to produce as much milk as possible. They are given shots of BST, bovine somatotrophin, a genetically engineered growth hormone, every other week.

The natural life span of a cow is twenty years. Dairy cows don't make it past seven. When they can't produce milk anymore, they are sent out to become hamburger for fast-food restaurants.

Seafood

I bet you didn't think that your wild Atlantic salmon was factory farmed. Fifty-thousand salmon are confined to a cage in the ocean. They are artificially colored, fattened on fish meal and oil, and given antibiotics and pesticides to reduce disease caused by such crowded living conditions. These thirty-inch salmon live in a space the size of a bathtub. Fish farming is the fastest growing form of food production in the world.

Producing animal products is a big business; it is an industry driven by the need for companies to make profits for their shareholders—just like any other business. The question of ethics here isn't about farmers treating animals cruelly, it is the system that pits profitability against animal welfare. And there is no way to avoid this—except by not eating animals in the first place. I bring to your awareness the incredible cruelty towards animals being produced to become food, not to cast judgment on the industry, but to give you one very good reason and motivating factor to consider turning away from eating animals and consuming a plant-based diet. If eating animals causes you ethical concern, there you have a good reason to think about the benefits of raw foods and healthier eating choices.

Ethical Arguments

Peter Singer, the famed animal rights activist, has put forward the marginal (newborns, senile) ethical argument for not eating animals. It goes like this: In order to conclude that only humans have the ethical right to live, they must have some property, P, that only humans have. There are properties that only humans have, but not all humans have them. Any property that all humans have, so do most animals. Therefore, we cannot conclude that only humans have the right to live. In other words, if newborns and senile people have the right to live, so do animals because they share the same properties.

Tom Regan, another intelligent writer on the topic of animal welfare, takes a different approach, the animal rights argument. By eating animals we are using them as a means to an end. Animals should be treated as ends in their own right. We should not be using animals, we should be respecting them. Why do humans have the right to life and animals don't? We give dogs and cats rights. What about whales? And dolphins? Horses? Why not cows and pigs? How can we choose some and not others? Can you not see the disparity of thought?

Ethical considerations comprise many reasons to be motivated to eat a vegan diet. A reasonably raw diet makes being a vegan easier.

Chapter 11

Douglas Graham and Natural Hygiene

*"Your instincts will reject or embrace each food on its merits—
that is, its appeals to your senses and palate—the only crite-
ria that guided our food selection in ages past."*

–Dr. Douglas Graham

As an approach to health, Natural Hygiene makes a lot of sense to me, rationally, intellectually, and instinctually. It draws upon our natural diet and instincts rather than what the human mind has determined appropriate to eat. In addition, the Natural Hygiene people, Douglas Graham in particular, take a strongly holistic approach to nutrition.

The holistic view held by Graham and the Natural Hygiene movement questions the value of isolating nutrients and their effect on health. Instead, we need to understand that health-promoting food comes packaged in a combination of elements more numerous than we can know. Micronutrients, many not even discovered yet, work in conjunction with each other. To isolate one vitamin or mineral and think that more or less of it will improve health is to ignore the natural package that nature has provided.

It is possible that we have only discovered about 10 percent of the plant nutrients in existence. This means that our health depends on a lot more than getting what we often think of as all our vitamins and minerals. For Graham, only a diet of whole foods will bring about a healthy body. Supplements may reduce and relieve symptoms, but only whole foods create health.

Eating By Design

Natural Hygiene makes the case, and a convincing one, that if you want to know what you should be eating, consider what you are designed to eat and what you would be eating naturally without cooking or altering the food. Douglas Graham, in his book *The 80/10/10 Diet,* points out that if you offer an animal all kinds of foods, in their natural state the animal will eat what is best for itself. The same should hold for humans.

In Graham's book he explains that if we were carnivores, we would relish the idea of catching an animal with our bare hands and eating it, entrails, fat, blood, bones, flesh, and all. Also, our bodies would be designed to eat other animals. (We've discussed this in a previous chapter.)

So much for being a carnivore. But what about the other "vores?" Herbivores forage on grass, weeds, and leaves. Unless that greenery is flavored with a great dressing, we do not find it particularly appealing. And it looks like it's by design we are not really made to eat them either, lacking the proper enzymes for digestion.

Likewise humans, unlike birds, are not all that attracted to grains, the seeds of grasses. We also don't get all that excited about eating raw tubers and legumes. Starches are just not very digestible by human beings.

How about milk? Surely dairy products do taste good, don't they? At least in the form of ice cream and cheese. True, but when was the last time you had the urge to suck on the breast of a wild animal, or even a cow or goat? That aside, milk contains casein, possibly one of the most active agents in the cause of cancer and heart disease. No other animal in the world drinks the milk of another animal.

Dr. Graham also takes a swipe at nuts and all high-fat plants. Humans have a difficult time digesting them and the fats are trapped in the intestine for long periods of time, causing all kinds of problems.

Everyone knows that humans are omnivores. We can eat just about anything. Yes, that may be the case, but a true omnivore thrives on everything just mentioned. As was stated before, being able to do something doesn't mean it is the best thing to do. Just because I can eat all of the above doesn't mean that I should.

So, given that all of these foods are unnatural to humans, what then are we to eat? Fruit. Fruit is the only food that in its natural state is appealing to us. And, best of all, we are designed perfectly to digest and utilize the plentiful carbohydrates in fruit. Fresh, ripe, raw fruit comes wrapped with digestible fiber, making sure that the fruit sugars enter our system gradually and for longer periods of time.

Humans, according to Graham, are frugivores, designed to live on fruit and tender greens. Think about it, fruits are the only food that all on its own can attract human beings. We see fruit growing and eat it just as it is. Certain greens have the ability to attract us also.

In my garden, I go for the tomatoes, a fruit. At the same time that we are naturally attracted to the sweetness in fruit, we just happen to be biologically designed to utilize and absorb the nutrients in fruits. This is the argument that really gets me. Of all the diets out there, the fruit diet makes the most sense logically and instinctually. We are naturally attracted to fruit and our bodies easily digest and utilize fruit.

Fruit: Facts, Fears, and Fats

Large quantities and even small quantities of fruit consumption are feared. Fruit is believed to cause high blood-sugar, which can cause diabetes, candida, chronic fatigue, and other illnesses. Eating fruit puts too much sugar into our blood. But Graham argues that fruit is not the problem, but fats.

Fruit, when eaten naturally, becomes a sugar in our body and then goes into the blood stream quickly and out of it into our cells, where it provides us nourishment. No problem. Primates eat enormous amounts of fruit in their natural habit.

The most significant contribution that Dr. Graham makes to our conversation here is this: a high-fat diet, one which nearly all of us have, makes it nearly impossible for fruit to get out of the blood stream and into our cells. Too much fat in the blood makes it difficult for fruit sugars to get out of our blood, causing high blood sugar.

Fatty food, by making a thin coating of fat on the blood-vessel walls, cell receptor sites, and sugar molecules themselves, in essence, gum up the whole works. The fats in our diets prevent the fruit that we eat from doing its job. And then fruit gets all the blame.

The thing is, we need the wonderful carbohydrates that fruit gives us to do most of the things we do. Without healthy carbs all sorts of disease and distress occur.

Fats take a long time to pass through the intestines, blood-stream, and into the cells. The whole process can take up to twenty-four hours. I used to think that I was safe if I ate fruit on an empty stomach. Wrong. My stomach may be empty, but my blood is not. It may still have fat floating around if I haven't gotten my consumption down to the level that Dr. Graham recommends.

If you remember anything at all from this chapter it is this: be very careful about how much fat you eat. Too much sabotages the essential work of fruit, and we all need lots of fruit. That is what we are designed to eat. So, if in the past you have had problems with fruit, it wasn't the fruit, it was probably the fat.

Balancing Calories: 80/10/10

The cornerstone of Dr. Graham's approach to excellent health is the need to balance the source of calories in one's diet. We get our calories from carbohydrates, proteins, and fats. The ratio of these three nutrients is vital to health, longevity, and energy. That ratio should be 80/10/10: a minimum 80 percent calories coming from carbohydrates, a maximum of 10 percent coming from protein, and a maximum 10 percent coming from fats.

This is the ratio that results when humans eat a mostly fruit diet. In the wild, primates like ourselves thrive on mostly fruits and tender greens. According to Graham, this ratio for chimps, bonobos, and orangutans (our closest cousins genetically), is 88/7/5.

Another argument for this ratio is that the longest living peoples approximate these percentages. The Abkhasians, the Vilcabambans, and the Hunza all consume around 70 percent of their calories in carbohydrates while obtaining about 15 percent from fat and 15 percent in protein.

Carbohydrates

Our bodies convert carbohydrates into simple sugars. Simple sugars, like glucose, are the fuels that run the engines of our bodies. We need carbohydrates for energy and health. Fresh fruits are the optimal source. The water-soluble fiber in fruit allows the sugars to be absorbed slowly into the blood stream.

There are other ways of obtaining carbohydrates, such as with grains, tubers, and legumes being the most obvious sources. Corn, rice, wheat, potatoes, carrots, beans, all make up a significant part of the American diet. In fact, these are the carbohydrates that most people think of when they think carbohydrates.

Many people are even aware that complex carbohydrates are better than processed. Whole wheat bread is better than white bread. There is a problem though. Grains, primarily wheat, cause all kinds of illnesses. Gluten intolerance is involved in the development of diabetes, arthritis, asthma, constipation, fibromyalgia, and autism.

Refined carbohydrates are essentially junk food; providing empty calories and leaving the body with no nutritional value. These empty calories simply accelerate the aging process.

Fresh, whole fruits provide carbohydrates without the problems. Easily digested and utilized, fruit should make up 80 percent of our calorie intake. Fruit is the least toxic and most nutritious source of energy for the human body. Human beings originated in the tropics, where we evolved eating tropical foods, fruits. This is what we are designed to eat, our natural diet.

Protein

The protein myth. A need created by the meat and dairy industry. Protein, we must have our protein. Where do I get my protein if I'm a vegan? The thing is: most of us eat way more than is good for us. We are not in danger of getting too little protein, but we are in danger of getting too much.

If anyone needs protein, it is a baby when growth is at its greatest. So how much protein does breast milk contain, the baby's natural source of nutrition? Only 6 percent of its calories come from protein. If we do not need a lot of protein as infants, why would we need more as adults? How much does the typical diet provide us? Around 15 percent, three times as much as we need. And the only reason it is as low as that is that the high protein foods we eat, meats and dairy products, have even more amounts of fat.

The overconsumption of protein is a serious problem. Too much protein causes too much acid to form in the human body. (This comes from acidic minerals: chlorine, phosphorus, sulfur.) The body wants the bloodstream to be in balance between acidity and alkalinity. Protein throws the balance off and so the body takes calcium, an alkaline mineral, from our bones and teeth, to restore this balance. This results in arthritis, osteoporosis, liver and kidney problems, autoimmune problems, and premature aging.

The thing is, animals are a bad source of protein anyhow. When we cook meat, we destroy half of the protein. The body has to break down what is left into amino acids. The body doesn't make protein from animal protein, but from amino acids. The advantage of getting protein from fruits and vegetables is that the body doesn't have to break down the protein; it is already there in the form of amino acids.

The best part of plant-based protein is that you can eat a lot less of it to get a lot more, more of what your body really needs. You are not adding more toxicity to your body in the form of hormones, antibiotics, and the drugs given to the animals that you eat. Eat your fruits and vegetables and you don't have to even think about protein again.

Fat

It is no surprise that a low fat diet is healthy. What is a surprise is how low low is. According to the USDA, 20 to 35 percent of our calories should come from fats. Dr. Graham recommends no more than 10 percent. He is supported in this by Dr. Dean Ornish, the Pritikin Longevity Center, and Dr. T. Colin Campbell in his book *The China Study*. The only reason the USDA recommends more is a result of the influence of the meat and dairy industries.

Besides causing weight and cholesterol problems, why should we limit our fat intake? Because fat in our blood makes it difficult for oxygen to reach our cells. It prevents fruits from delivering the sugars that we need for energy and healthy bodily functions.

If you are going to consume fat, it should come from whole foods and not oil. Oil is stripped of the fiber which keeps fats from going rancid. Oil is pure fat. It is best to get your fats from fresh nuts, seeds, and avocados. Oil is a processed food providing empty calories.

Dr. Graham takes a chapter of his book to warn that many people who eat only raw food eat way too much fat. When people convert to raw food diets, they tend to eat a lot of food with fat in order to feel satisfied. Many raw food recipes use nuts and seeds to mimic cooked foods. This negates all the benefits of eating raw foods. Also, by eating so many fatty foods they end up not eating as much fruit as they need to. Instead of feeling energized and healthy, their bodies become clogged up with too much fat. (Many vegetarians are not all that healthy because they consume a lot of dairy products.)

Making It Work

Natural Hygiene and the 80/10/10 diet are the most radical of all the approaches to raw food. They are the most difficult to implement. Since they require the reduction and elimination of so much protein and fat, a person trying to eat this way will starve and find it nearly impossible to do unless they significantly increase the amount of fruit eaten.

I believe that Natural Hygiene may be the healthiest way to go. Fats do hinder fruits from providing the fuel that our bodies need. Protein, besides causing all kinds of problems with too much acidity in the blood and the depletion of calcium, is a major factor in heart disease and cancer, as proven by the China Study. And fruits and vegetables are what we humans are designed to eat.

There is one problem in this. Getting rid of fats and proteins and living on only fruits and vegetables is an incredibly difficult task. How does one do it? According to the Natural Hygiene forums and testimonials it is done by gradually increasing the amount of fruit consumed at every meal. Always eat your fruit first so it doesn't get stuck fermenting behind the heavier foods. Eat much more than you think you should. Successful people on this type of diet typically eat two pounds of fruit at a meal. They also eat a whole head of lettuce at dinnertime.

There is one other word of caution I want to mention. There is great controversy in the raw food movement regarding Natural Hygiene. While at the Raw Spirit Festival in Arizona, I met a number of people who had been on the diet and had health problems and had to go back to a more conventional form of raw foodism. At the same time others swear by it. All I can say is try it and see how you feel. Whether you incorporate the whole 80/10/10 diet or not, the ideas in this program are valuable.

The Best of Douglas Graham

The most important lessons from the writing and research of Dr. Graham are these: 1.) make fruit the central and largest part of your diet 2.) seriously keep your consumption of fats to a minimum 3.) avoid meats and dairy because they contain too much protein and fat. We need to eat a lot more fruit than we think. We probably are eating a lot more fat than we should. And a vegan diet is best because vegans do not stuff their bodies with animal protein, toxic hormones, and body-clogging fats.

While following Graham's 80/10/10 diet may be hard to accomplish, at least seeing it as a goal to reach, or an incentive, is better than being ignorant of the ideal. I could see a time in my life, especially as I get older, where a light diet, based on easily digested fruits, would be so attractive. The less our bodies have to work on digesting food, the more energy we have left over to live our lives to the fullest.

Further Reading:

The 80/10/10 Diet. Dr. Douglas Graham. 2006. FoodnSport Press.

Chapter 12

Gabriel Cousens
and Conscious Eating

"The art of conscious eating lies in creating an individualized diet that reflects and supports one's realization of the highest state of awareness, as well as one's need to function in the world of everyday life."

—GABRIEL COUSENS

Gabriel Cousens has an M.D., an M.D. (H), and a D.D. He is a psychiatrist, acupuncturist, Reiki Master, medical researcher, Ayurvedic practitioner, and author. He is also the founder and director of the Tree of Life Rejuvenation Center in Patagonia, Arizona. Dr. Cousens has been a raw food vegan since 1983.

When it comes to the science of living foods and health, there isn't anyone more qualified to make statements and recommendations. Besides his medical background Cousens has spent numerous years studying spirituality with indigenous teachers (both Native Americans and Indians), and he is an ordained Essene teacher.

Self-composting

Taking a medical doctor's approach, Cousens' search for extraordinary health begins with a close look at blood. He begins by drawing on the research performed by Antoine Bechamp in the early 1900's, and concludes that the human body's blood is not so much a liquid as it is a flowing tissue. Looking closer at this system, Bechamp theorized that microscopic and colloidal elements, smaller than cells, were living in our bodies and fermenting sugar in our blood.

This microscopic digestion produced toxins, mycotoxins. These toxins are the forerunners of degenerative disease—illness. When the natural fermentation process speeds up due to excess sugar in the system, these microzymas turn into bacteria, yeast, fungus, and mold. And that is when health degenerates.

Acid foods, along with acid thoughts, environmental toxins, lack of oxygen, all play a part in distorting what Cousens calls the "subtle organizing energy field." This energy exists in the space between cells, which we know is relatively large. The body is continually recycling itself. In a healthy state this goes on undisturbed. But when fermentation begins, the body is essentially composting itself and a cycle of degeneration initiates, allowing chronic disease to get a foothold.

Cousens teaches that a low-sweet, live-food, non-acidic diet can turn off the self-composting process. This means eliminating junk food, refined foods, and canned foods. We need to remove the causes of yeast and fungus. That means steroids, antibiotics, birth control pills, alcohol, and animal products. These acid-promoting foods create the conditions for mold and fungus to turn healthy blood into oxygen-deprived clumps. Not a good system for delivering oxygen and nutrients throughout the body.

In the end we are left with a greatly weakened immune system, a pre-cancerous condition, as Cousens writes. The results: allergies, fatigue, depression, anxiety, colds, poor mental capabilities, diabetes, heartburn, vaginal yeast infections, joint pain, asthma, and food cravings to name a few.

The Culprits

There are certain foods that contain large quantities of mycotoxins and fungus. Anything with a high sugar content contributes to self-composting. Other foods include animal fats, dairy products, mushrooms, table salt, soy sauce, microwaved foods, and saturated vegetable oils.

According to Cousens' theory, foods high in sugar should be avoided more than any other type of food. This includes not only processed white sugar but also fruits with a high glycemic index. Sugar substitutes such as corn sugar, sorbital, maple sugar, and honey are to be avoided. High sugar fruits include melons, bananas, mangoes, pineapple, papaya, kiwi, and apricots. Dried fruits are high in sugar content. White flour, white rice, and white potatoes raise blood glucose. Apple juice is the most dangerous of all because it contains a mycotoxin that research shows to cause mammary tumors in mice.

The central concern of Cousens' diet is to eliminate foods that stimulate the production of yeast, fungi, and molds. High sugar foods and fruit are at the top of the list, grains come in second. This is because they are stored for long periods of time and begin to ferment. Non-stored grains, such as quinoa, buckwheat, millet, spelt, and wild rice, are not a health hazard.

Grains are acid-forming, not a good thing. Grains also contain coarse non-soluble fiber, which while being good for adding bulk to the diet, is an irritant to the colon. Grain causes food to move too rapidly through the intestines, reducing nutrient absorption.

The flour used to bake many products has been sitting around for more than a year, breeding mold and fungus. And we know that the government allows a certain percentage of insect parts and rodent fecal matter.

Animal products are another breeding ground for mycotoxins. First, animals are fed fungally infected feed. Secondly, we know that meats and dairy acidify the blood. Third, meals consisting of animal products contain more than a million times the pathogenic microorganisms found in vegan meals.

Other foods high in mycotoxins and fungi are corn, peanuts, cashews, oats, yeast (baker's yeast, brewers yeast, and nutritional yeast), caffeine, tobacco, and coffee. All cooked foods should be avoided.

Keep in mind that this composting process thrives on sugar, which drives our food cravings. While sugar is found in the obvious places like sweets and sweet fruits, processed flours and grains are easily converted into sugars. **The fungus living in our bodies creates the**

food cravings that many of us suffer from. Eliminate the fungus and we eliminate the cravings.

The Optimal Diet

While no single diet is best for everyone, there are key principles to healthy eating. First, eat organically grown food if at all possible. This will reduce consumption of genetically modified organisms and toxic chemicals. These foods contain more vitamins and minerals, taste better, and have more phytochemicals. They are also better for the environment. At Cousens' Tree of Life Center they practice what is called Nature Farming, where they attempt to build the soil and compost exclusively with plant materials, modeling natural forests and prairies.

The second aspect of a healthy diet is that it restricts calories. There is a great deal of evidence showing that longevity is linked to living on significantly fewer calories than we are used to. This is born out in the long-living peoples such as the Hunzas, the Abkhasians, and the Vilcabamban Indians. They live on roughly half the calories of the typical American.

My first thought about this is that I'd have to starve myself and I'll be hungry all the time. However, according to Cousens' research, and others, the reason we consume the calories that we do is that cooking destroys more than 50 percent of the nutrients in our foods. So we crave more food, we have to eat more food to give our bodies what it needs. By switching to a live-food, raw diet, we will eat less because we will want less. This is one of the most significant reasons for converting as much of your diet to live-food as possible.

Finally, the optimal diet, according to the Cousens program, is primarily one that includes low-glycemic fruits, vegetables, nuts, seeds, sea vegetables, and algae. Of course, these are all prepared without cooking. Low-glycemic fruits include blueberries, strawberries, goji berries, grapefruit, cherries, and lemons. Moderately glycemic fruits are allowed also, these include oranges, apples, peaches, pears, and plums. Fruits containing high quantities of sugar, such as melons, bananas, pineapple, grapes, mango, kiwi, and most dried fruits, should be avoided or eaten in moderation.

Vegetable fruits like avocados, tomatoes, cucumbers, and zucchini are good to eat along with all vegetables (especially green leafy ones), nuts and seeds, and sea vegetables (dulse, nori, kelp). Carrots are good, as well as fresh coconut (both water and meat).

Conscious Eating

In Cousens' tome *Conscious Eating* he offers his insights into a more spiritual approach to eating, health, and nutrition. He writes that conscious eating is being aware of how our food affects us holistically—body, mind, emotions, and spirit. We become aware of how our food choices affect other human beings, animals, and the entire planet. Conscious eating involves an awareness of the Divine.

Cousens' approach to conscious eating expands nutritional awareness to include elements of the Hindu health care system known as

Ayurveda, naturopathy, homeopathy, and acupuncture. Yoga, meditation, breathing exercises, and other spiritual practices have a place in acquiring a more healthy way of eating.

Conscious eating is the act of individualizing one's diet. Each of us, being unique, must find a diet that works for ourselves. There is no one diet that applies to everyone. Creating a diet that works for us is helped by trial-and-error, experimenting, and using our intelligence to find the foods and their combinations most helpful to healthful living. In presenting a broad range of the most successful raw food leaders, I have attempted in this book to provide a sampling so that you could be exposed to a number of paths to healthy eating and find one or more, or a combination, that is best suited to your needs.

It is helpful when considering our diet to honor not only the needs of our body, but also one that promotes a clear mind and unfettered spirit. We want a diet that is in harmony with nature, considerate of animals, and contributes to peace on the planet. Does it make sense to add to the misery of sentient beings, both human and animal? Can we expect health when we do this? We will reap what we sow, especially when it comes to food, the very most basic element of life.

For Additional Readings on Conscious Eating:

Conscious Eating. Gabriel Cousens, M.D. 2000. North Atlantic Books.

Rainbow Green Live-Food Cuisine. Gabriel Cousens, M.D. and the Tree of Life Café Chefs. 2003. North Atlantic Books.

Chapter 13

Getting Started

"The secret of getting started is breaking your complex overwhelming tasks into small manageable tasks, and then starting on the first one."

—Mark Twain

You want to change your diet. You know that eating animals is not a good thing, for you, for them, or for the planet. You know now that cooking foods might not be a good thing. It makes sense that living beings live better on living foods. But you absolutely do not want to give up the foods that you love. In fact, you really don't want to make any drastic changes to your life at all. Don't feel bad—that makes you like everyone else.

That is why I am going to help you get started with this chapter. I am going to show you a painless and fairly simple way to get on the path to great health, good karma, and a cleaner planet. Above all else remember this—never, ever, ever, think about giving up the food that you love. We are not going to try go give up anything. Trying to stop eating foods does not work. We are going add things to your life. And this you can do.

First Things First

The first thing to add to your diet is a delicious green smoothie. You want to start your day with the perfect food on an empty stomach—fruit. We always want to eat fruit on an empty stomach, otherwise it gets stuck behind slower digesting foods that cause the fruit not to be absorbed very well. Eat your fruit first.

It is important to experiment a little when you begin making your smoothies. We all have different tastes and likes. Make your smoothie delicious for you. If your first attempt isn't great, change it around the next time. Put in fruits that you love, try different combinations. Make your smoothie so good that you can't wait to have it. I make mine so good that I have to pace myself otherwise I will drink it down too fast, and I have them everyday.

You want to put a little liquid into the blender first. Maybe some water, fresh squeezed orange juice, or coconut water (my favorite). Then put in your fruit (pineapple goes well with oranges and berries), blend it up. In the beginning add only a small amount of dark leafy greens. Two or three kale or romaine leafs, or a handful of spinach. Later on you can add more; I put in twice that amount and cannot taste it.

Put some frozen fruit in last. I like strawberries and blueberries. I have found that the best fruits for smoothies are oranges, pineapples, bananas, blueberries, watermelon, mangoes, and strawberries. As a treat, a few times a week I throw in the water and meat of a young Thai coconut. Your smoothie should be delicious, refreshing, and keep you full way past lunchtime. I usually make a quart and I am not hungry until one or two o'clock in the afternoon. (There is a video on my blog—reasonablyraw.blogspot.com—showing how I make my smoothies. And there are lots of other videos on youtube demonstrating many other possibilities. Just type in "green smoothies" in the search.)

Remember, you do not have to have an early breakfast. Most of us think we have to eat first thing in the morning, but that is not true. It is actually healthier to eat, or drink it, later on. This gives your body more time to digest yesterday's food. And you'll have more energy early on an empty stomach. If you are eating healthier, you most likely will begin sleeping better and not wake up hungry.

Your Tastes Change

Once you have made green smoothies a regular part of your life, something interesting happens. Now remember, you have not thought about giving anything up at all. You are just adding smoothies. But your body is changing. You are ingesting and your body is utilizing nutrients that you haven't had before—even if you thought you were eating healthily. Your body begins to feel better and very subtly starts asking for more of this good stuff. The cravings for meats and processed foods diminish just a little, but enough for you to notice. Now you are going to make another easy little addition to your eating habits—a really big salad before dinner.

Green leafy vegetables are, along with fruits, the key to health. You have gotten a small but potent dose of them in your morning smoothie, and now you are going to perfect that with a wonderful evening salad. No iceberg lettuce here, only the dark leafy kind. And not a little bowl but a good dinner-sized salad.

Suppose you don't like salad. No problem. The secret to a great salad is finding a dressing that you love. Again, experiment until your mouth waters at the thought of the big salad you are going to have tonight. I am a very fortunate man; my daughter Gina has given me four recipes, which I include in the back of this book, that I totally love. I rotate them around, as I am inclined. Some of them I also use as a veggie dip for broccoli, peppers, carrots, and celery.

Do whatever it takes to love your big salad. Keep searching until you have at least three or four dressings that you can't live without. Make the dressings yourself at home with fresh ingredients, never use the store bought. Homemade dressings are so much better.

By adding a green smoothie for breakfast and a large salad before dinner, you have given your body an incredible amount of nutrients. You are feeding your body real food. Once again you will experience a subtle change in your food desires. Not that you will want to give up all your old foods. Years and years of eating animals and processed foods are ingrained into your body and psyche. However, you will find that while those foods still strongly dominate your mind, your body is feeling different. You will have less and less physical craving for dead food. And you still have not tried to give anything up.

The addition of a green smoothie and a big salad is really not a big thing. No one has asked you to give up anything. There is no pain here.

It doesn't get much easier. There is no diet to go on. No calories to count. You are naturally going to make better food choices because your body is feeling better.

Raw Dishes

Okay, you've made it this far, what's next? First you get more recipes for raw food dishes. Not a lot, but four or five that you can use for lunch or dinner. I suggest buying a DVD demonstrating raw food preparation; this is much easier than reading from a book and much more inspiring. For me just one DVD gave me the confidence to experiment on my own. (Alissa Cohen's book and DVD Living On Live Food are excellent.) Or you can go on youtube.com and you can find just about anything there for free. The recipes are amazing.

Several of my favorite dinner time foods are guacamole, cauliflower mashed potatoes, Cohen's crepes, and a mock tuna salad. I've learned to make a raw marinara sauce. Often I will just mash up an avocado and add a heaping spoonful of the marinara sauce, and I've got a delicious guacamole. It takes all of two minutes to prepare.

It is absolutely essential to take the time to learn a few good dishes; otherwise you will never get past always having to have a cooked dinner. Once you learn a few recipes you will be amazed at how good and filling they are.

The biggest weapon I have in my arsenal is my durian ice cream and mousse. Durian is a tropical fruit that comes from Southeast Asia. You can buy it at most Asian markets. Durian is the perfect substitute for anything creamy, milky, or custardy. I use the durian as a base for my chocolate ice cream, and if I don't want to be bothered with using the ice cream maker, I let the ingredients sit in the refrigerator and it becomes a mousse. Warning—durian has a unique flavor and smell and it takes two or three times eating it to get used to its specialness.

A Second Smoothie

Another step towards a more raw and healthful diet is the option to add a second smoothie for lunch. I find this convenient and enjoyable. The breakfast smoothie gives you a great shot of fruit to begin your day, along with a little bit of greens. Why not a second smoothie? Blending foods certainly makes it easier on the digestive system, allowing you more energy to do want you want to do. The key here is to make this smoothie taste significantly different from the first one.

I make my afternoon smoothie into a "superfood" smoothie. It tastes totally different from my morning one; it's more like a shake. I use a base of water and bananas. I add in maca, hemp seed, spirulina, dulse or kelp powder, coconut butter, and agave. Then, most important of all, one heaping tablespoon of raw cacao powder for a delicious chocolate flavor. This tastes like a chocolate milk shake. My smoothie, filled with superfoods, powers me till dinnertime. And even by then I'm not all that hungry after feeding my body with so many absorbable nutrients. That is the key to eliminating overeating and eating junk food.

With my fruit smoothie and superfood smoothie, I have found it so easy to stay raw all day. That leaves me with plenty of options for dinner. The best thing is that I have more energy and I have given my body so many nutrients. Both of my smoothies taste so good that I absolutely look forward to drinking them. And they are both easily portable. I pour my second one into a quart mason jar, put it in a small cooler, and take it with me.

Go Slowly – Have Fun

If you focus only on adding healthy foods to your diet and not taking anything away, I promise that you will succeed. Approach raw eating from the perspective of adding healthy habits and not trying to deny yourself the foods you think that you cannot live without. Do not even worry about it. Little by little you will find that your tastes change. Ever so slightly you will notice that you don't need or want to eat as much meat, or fish, or dairy. How easy could this be? As your smoothies and salads and raw dishes nourish your body, it will crave less and less the dead foods. This can be a totally painless process. (The only pain comes when you try too hard to make yourself stop eating things that for years you have been used to eating and found pleasure in them. As strange as it sounds you will find great pleasure in fruits and salads.)

This does not mean there will not be times when you feel miserable and want that greasy burger and fries. You will take steps backwards. This is the human condition. It is all part of our journey. So, while we can make healthy living easier, we cannot make it easy. Sometimes we have to hoe the garden, pull the weeds, water the tomatoes.

I have found that by reading books on raw foods, visiting raw food web sites, talking to friends about their successes and difficulties, I get more motivated, more inspired. The more living foods I put in my body, the better I feel and the less I want to eat junk foods. I sleep better, I work better, I play better. So, be good to yourself. Be patient, slowly add smoothies and salads and raw entrees to your diet, and you will wake up one day feeling so light, so cheerful, and so refreshed, you will wonder why everyone doesn't live like this.

Chapter 14

The Change Process: Becoming Raw

"If nothing ever changed, there'd be no butterflies."

–Author Unknown

"It is not the strongest of the species that survive, nor the most intelligent, but the one most responsive to change."

–Author unknown, commonly misattributed to Charles Darwin

"If you would attain to what you are not yet, you must always be displeased by what you are. For where you are pleased with yourself there you have remained."

–Saint Augustine

You think you want to become a raw vegan. You want to try eating more fruits and raw vegetables. You want to convince your friends and family that raw food will make them healthier. You want to change.

You know your past failures.

It is not easy to change; if it were everyone would be just the way they want to be. Do you know anyone who is satisfied with who they are, who doesn't want to change some aspect of themselves? Change is a lot of hard work and commitment. I am here to tell you that anything worth having, including excellent health, comes at a price. So don't complain, just reach into your pocket and pull out your wallet. But, there is hope, and it can be made easier.

One of the biggest obstacles that we face when we want to make changes in our lives is to underestimate the difficulty in changing and not understanding the change process. This all too easily leads to frustration, pain, and the end of putting into place the changes we want to make. This does not need to happen.

I have included this chapter on change so that you may find it easier to implement what you have learned in this book and be able to share your new insights with others in a more thoughtful and intelligent way. Attaining a healthy, energetic body, saving our planet, and reducing the suffering of other sentient beings is a sacred and noble undertaking; it deserves a serious and well-planned attempt. I hope to increase your chances of success by sharing with you my research on the change process; together we will explore the stages and processes of change.

The Stages of Change

There has been a great deal of research committed to the understanding of how people are able to successfully change their behavior. Much of the study in this area is focused on behavior involving drug abuse, smoking, and mental health. But the lessons learned there are fully applicable to changing eating patterns. In this chapter I draw from the work of James O. Prochaska, Ph.D., professor of psychology at the University of Rhode Island. His book, *Changing For Good,* describes one of the most successful programs for implementing personal change ever developed.

"Things do not change; we change."

–HENRY DAVID THOREAU

In the raw food world, Victoria Boutenko says that we should go cold turkey to change our diet. And David Wolfe likes to encourage raw food progress by suggesting that we do it "little by little"; and that we should focus on adding raw food into our diets and not to be concerned with giving foods up. Who is to say which way is best?

We need to take into consideration that change is seldom a linear process, most of the time it is cyclical, spiral, and circular. If you are a "normal" human being, you will most likely take two steps forward and one step back. Sometimes you may take two steps back and one step forward. That is the way we learn and grow. There is no sense in fighting it, but it does help a lot if you are aware that relapse and setbacks are common and that you expect your journey to health to be a spiral one.

We become who we want to be by working, consciously or unconsciously, on life problems and finding their solutions. Change happens through a series of stages. The reason that understanding the stages of change is important is that each stage requires a different tool, demands a different approach. Each stage of change has its own process of change, as we will see shortly.

The six clearly-defined stages of change are: precontemplation, contemplation, preparation, action, maintenance, and termination. We will be discussing each stage and its corresponding process shortly. Some of the processes that match certain stages of change are: consciousness-raising, social liberation, emotional arousal, self-reevaluation, commitment, countering, and environmental control. What I want to stress now is that by understanding each stage, by determining where we are (or where someone whom we want to help make changes is), we can match the appropriate efforts and processes to work through that stage to the next one and eventually reach our goal of healthful eating.

The experiences at each stage are predictable for all people. Each stage has its own task to be completed before moving on to the next. Warning! It is possible to get stuck in one stage. However, if we understand the stages and processes useful in each one, we will move through more quickly and easily. You will experience less guilt, shame, anxiety, and pain.

Precontemplation

The precontemplation stage is characterized by denial. There is no problem as far as one who is in precontemplation is concerned. The food they eat, what it does to them, the environment, the suffering caused, is not even on their radar screens. Total oblivion. A person in the precontemplation stage will deny having a problem, even if it is brought into their awareness. If they do not totally deny the problem they will at least minimize it. "I eat lots of fruits and vegetables, and have only chicken and fish for protein. What more can I do?"

When I was told that my cholesterol was 242, I first wondered how that could be. My doctor said that if I couldn't get it down by eating better I'd have to take medication. I said I already am eating better. (This was before I started eating raw.) Then I went online to satisfy myself that 242 wasn't all that bad after all and it was just the drug companies trying to sell more drugs. It wasn't until my blood pressure became hypertensive that I finally admitted to myself that I had a problem.

"It is impossible for a man to learn what he thinks he already knows."

—EPICTETUS

Besides resistance, precontemplators are often demoralized. Since there is no possibility for change, they feel hopeless. "How can one live on just raw food? Where will I get my protein? What is the use in living without the enjoyment of a good steak, or lobster, or hamburger?"

Most people, when approached with the proposition that a raw food diet would be good for them, and the planet as well, will be in this stage. (You, the reader, are most likely not. If you are reading this book you and have gotten this far, you are at least at the contemplation stage.) What to do?

There are two processes of change that work for helping the person in the precontemplation stage—consciousness-raising and social liberation. (Yikes, what the heck is social liberation?) The goal of consciousness-raising is to increase information about the self and the problem. The goal of social liberation is to increase social alternatives to the old ways of living and eating.

Consciousness-raising

You have discovered the joy of raw food and the health that comes with it. You want to share this with friends and family. Heck, you want to save the planet. Why not? So, how do you do this? First, assume that everyone you meet is a precontemplator—at least as far as raw food goes.

In psychology we talk about making the unconscious conscious. Mental health is all about this and increasing awareness. (It is no coincidence that meditation practices and spiritual development also center around consciousness-raising. I strongly believe that our eating habits affect our spirituality.) When we increase the level of awareness, we are bringing new information to ourselves and others, increasing the possibility of making better choices regarding what needs to be changed.

"Change is hard because people overestimate the value of what they have—and underestimate the value of what they may gain by giving that up."

—JAMES BELASCO AND RALPH STAYER, *FLIGHT OF THE BUFFALO*

In short, in this stage we are increasing knowledge about nutrition, the differences between cooked food and raw food, the health benefits, the joy of eating raw food (and all the available options); we become informed or we inform others. This is the goal.

The first step in change at this level is to bring into awareness the defenses of precontemplation—denial, minimization, rationalization, projection, and internalization. The second step is to simply provide information about what happens when we eat the Standard American Diet and what happens when we begin eating more and more raw food.

That being said, it is essential not to rush anyone, including yourself, toward action. The research on successful change makes it clear that change must proceed through the stages. A raised consciousness about raw food does not mean we are ready to change. It means we *may* be ready to *think* about change. So let's be patient with ourselves.

Social Liberation

Part of sharing the newfound joys of raw food involves sharing the alternatives that are available. The idea of just eating raw food sounds so utterly boring. I remember meeting my first raw food person while I was away at a colloquium beginning my Ph. D. studies. I thought, "What in the world is there for him to possibly eat?" Eating raw was the last thing that I wanted to do.

However, several years later, along comes my daughter Gina. She was the first person to tell me about the benefits (consciousness-raising) of raw food and the first person to invite me to a raw potluck dinner party (social liberation). Gina made me a number of tasty raw food treats. At the potluck dinner I was able to experience and enjoy foods that were totally satisfying and were every bit as tasty as the old cooked foods I was so used to eating.

Besides the excellent food at these raw dinners, I enjoyed talking to other people about their experiences. Being part of a small community like this also makes starting out on the raw journey seem not so crazy. Talking to my daughter nearly every day about some aspect of being raw helps to keep me motivated.

Contemplation

We reach the contemplation stage when we realize that we have a problem. In some way we become aware that maybe the food we are eating is not all that healthy. The evidence is too strong to deny, or minimize, or rationalize away. We may have a health crisis. Or, we might see something positive that awakens us. For me, seeing my daughter and son-in-law after they had been on a raw diet for one month, made me stop and think—they were literally glowing! (Even today, the sight of my daughter looking so healthy and beautiful makes me smile and thank God for the raw food movement.)

Openness is the essence of contemplation. We become curious. However, while we may want to change, there remains resistance and ambivalence—fear of the unknown. There is a sense of wishing we could change, but not quite enough motivation to change. Sometimes we try to change prematurely, and that can lead to failure and guilt.

The key to contemplation is that the contemplator begins to acknowledge that there is a problem. Faced with the facts of my high blood pressure, I had to admit that something was not right. It is in the admitting process that the emotions kick in, and that is the necessary requirement to begin work in this stage. This leads us to the next process of change—emotional arousal.

Emotional Arousal

Emotional arousal is the impetus to push along the change process. It is the motivating force, the fuel that gets us ready to prepare and then take action. For many people, coming face to face with a health crisis jump-starts our interest in raw food. Nothing gets you emotionally aroused liked pain, the fear of death, or even just looking fat. The loss of youthful energy can inspire people to consider making changes in their lives.

"Be the change you want to see in the world."

–Mahatma Gandhi

Fear is not often a good motivator—it is easily dismissed by our defenses—so I do not recommend focusing on that. Instead, become involved emotionally with the positive side of changing your diet. The thought of losing weight, fitting into better looking clothes and, having more energy can be inspiring. I like to think about not supporting the meat and dairy industries, reducing the suffering of animals, polluting the planet less. The feel of my clothes and a slimmer body motivate me still.

In a sense, emotional arousal is consciousness-raising but on a deeper, more personal level. At this stage it might be good to watch movies and documentaries about the effects of an animal-based diet or the benefits of eating raw food. Even better, go to a raw food festival. Emotional arousal comes with whatever motivates you. Consciousness-raising will only take you so far; if you remain at the intellectual level you will never take action. Learn how to become motivated.

Self-reevaluation

Self-reevaluation also involves the emotions and deep personal feelings. It involves an honest look at the life you are living and determining if how you are living corresponds to your personal values. Self-reevaluation is a time for asking tough questions. Do I really want to contribute to the suffering of animals? Is that the kind of person I am? Do I really want to contribute to the unnecessary waste of natural resources and the harming of this planet? Is eating so much cooked food worth an early death, or a life with barely enough energy to get by?

"It is not necessary to change. Survival is not mandatory."

–W. EDWARDS DEMING

If we are in the contemplative stage we will use this time to consider the pros and cons of making the change. What is the cost of change? Some of the cons of increasing the consumption of raw food are: having to learn new ways of preparing meals, dealing with temptations at restaurants, not eating all of the foods we have grown up loving and, having to think about and plan meals in advance.

What, then, are the benefits and rewards of change? Some of the pros are: having more energy, a better physical appearance, clearer thinking, less pain from disease or worry about getting an illness. These are all ideas that arise in the contemplative stage of change. Considering these tough questions will prepare one for the time of action that is coming.

But more than looking at the pros and cons, we take stock of ourselves and honestly examine who we are and if we are living in accordance with our values. This need not involve beating ourselves up for what we have been doing. Instead, we can look at the future and see how we can make our lives better. We think about the consequences of eating differently.

Preparation

You have decided that it is time to change. Contemplation has brought you to the point where enough is enough; you are committed to making changes in your life. Hold on, admit it, there is a little ambivalence, you are not totally sure you can do this, but you are ready to try.

Research shows that it is best to do a little planning, even develop a scheme for action, be clear in your mind what to expect and how to succeed. Before jumping into the raw food world, be prepared. Your consciousness is raised, you are emotionally involved, now you must remove any ambivalence so that your commitment will be firm.

You are at the intersection of contemplation and action. Plan how you will succeed. Read more books on raw food. Find out the pitfalls, explore interesting recipe books, stock up on delicious raw foods and spices. But most of all, be certain of your commitment.

Commitment

As I said before, change is hard, very hard. If it were easy, everyone would be living wonderful lives—and most people are not. The most important concept and idea that you must get into your head is this— make eating healthily the most important thing in your life. Make change a priority. Think about all of the benefits and let them motivate you. Nothing is more important than your health, and making this change comes first.

Some of the steps of preparation and commitment involve going public (tell people your intentions). Nothing helps commitment like stepping out on a limb and exposing yourself. Prepare yourself mentally. I am a big fan of meditation and relaxation practices.

"It doesn't work to leap a twenty-foot chasm in two ten-foot jumps."

—AMERICAN PROVERB

Probably more than anything, I believe reading books provides more information about how to develop a plan of action than anything else. Just reading this book will make a major difference in your chances of success. Closely related to this are online articles and online discussion groups. I highly endorse the yahoo group rawfood. (Rawfood – Raw Food for Health and Happiness)

Action

We have stopped denying that we have a problem with the foods we eat. We have learned that consuming more raw foods will make us and the planet healthier. We are sick and tired of being sick and tired. We have a plan to change what and how we eat. We are ready for action.

In the action stage we actually change our behavior. We change our surroundings and make the move. This is where we really have to be ready for problems. But, by having educated yourself about the stages of change, you will be better prepared to deal with the inevitable setbacks and frustrations.

"In order to change we must be sick and tired of being sick and tired."

—AUTHOR UNKNOWN

Remember, the action stage is only one stage in the process of changing and benefiting from a raw food diet. Also, our actions are only part of the process; we continue to change our levels of awareness, we involve our emotions, our thoughts, our self-images. Change is a cyclical means of becoming someone new.

The fact that you are aware of the dangers inherent in trying to change does not guarantee that you will be successful. In fact, I can guarantee that you will curse the day that you ever heard about raw foods. So, beware of taking the action step lightly, change costs; there is no easy way to improve your diet. That being said, here are several more processes that will help.

Countering

Countering is simply substituting healthy responses for poor behavior. It is also the most important tool in your change process toolbox. It does no good to give up eating animals and cooking most of your food if you do not have something to replace those behaviors. Countering is finding substitutes and healthy replacements. Here are a few countering techniques:

1. Relaxation and yoga, meditation and prayer.
2. Exercise. This is the most important thing you can do to succeed.
3. Active diversion. Find something else to do: read, walk, make love, etc.
4. Counterthinking. Change your way of thinking. Get positive.
5. Assertiveness. Don't let other people keep you in your old way of eating.

Who would think that meditation and prayer would play a part in changing behavior? Certainly all of the people who have been helped by the 12-Step Programs. I am not sure what comes first, eating healthfully or a new interest in spirituality. Either way, the two seem to go hand in hand. Eating more raw food has improved my meditation practice and my meditation practice has helped me improve my eating habits. Maybe both help me to see things more clearly. Whatever it is, there seems to be a symbiotic relationship going on between these two aspects of my life.

Meditation is also an aid in counterthinking, as it gives you the tools to eliminate negative thoughts and replace them with positive. It is all about becoming more self-aware of who we are and what we are doing.

Exercise is essential to good health—physical and mental. (By the way, if trying to change your behavior makes you despair, research shows that vigorous exercise is the one thing that can be guaranteed to cure your depression.) I run five miles every morning before breakfast. I would not think of not running. I cannot imagine being healthy without a serious exercise program. Make it a top priority in your life.

Active diversion is simple: keep yourself busy, make your life interesting—otherwise you will eat poorly out of boredom. Watching television is not a good choice here.

Assertiveness is simply taking charge of your own life and not letting others get in the way. External pressures have a way of helping us to slip back into our old ways. I am sure that at first you will give in, but after a few times of being frustrated by the results, you will let your emotions give you the strength you need to assert what you want.

Environmental Control

Countering is an internal process; environmental control is external. Do you want to eat healthy food? Throw out the chips; remove all the food that you have chosen not to eat from your house. Replace the old recipe books with new ones on raw uncooking.

When we change our surroundings, we make it easier to change our actions. I find that if I have only healthy food in the house, I eat healthy food. If I eliminate junk food, at night if I have a craving for something processed and sugary, I will not get in my car to go out and buy something. Instead, if all I have is fruit, and if I'm really hungry and not just bored, I'll eat that instead.

It is not cheating to modify your environment, it is smart planning. Why rely on willpower? Avoidance is perfectly acceptable when you are trying to change. If you were giving up alcohol would you keep beer in the refrigerator? Avoidance is not limited to objects; you can avoid people and places, too.

Maintenance

In the beginning we are really excited about raw foods and the changes in how we feel now that we are eating more healthily. It is an exciting time. We may be motivated by fear; we've had a health scare. We may be encouraged because we are losing weight fast. We might be experiencing renewed energy. Whatever it is, we are emotionally charged.

But the war is not won yet. We are only halfway there. To make change permanent we have to understand that this is a long-term effort. The changes we have made to our lifestyle need to be sustained, and it takes time for them to be firmly established. We need to build on what we started with.

First, realize that you will still be vulnerable. Habits take time to become ingrained. If you slip, do not beat yourself up, just start over again tomorrow.

Second, don't forget to use the processes that got you here in the first place. Use all the strategies from contemplation to action. Keep up with the exercise, meeting with like-minded people, read, join a yahoo raw foods group, go to a festival or retreat.

Third, keep controlling your environment. Avoid people, places, and things that will make it easier to fall back into poor eating habits.

This is not a sign of weakness, but one of intelligence.

Lastly, remind yourself every day, as I do, that this is the most important thing you can do for yourself. Health, energy, and fitness have to be worked at, they do not just happen. Let your mind help you. Cultivate consciousness.

Slips, Relapses, and Recycling

It is going to happen, you might as well be prepared. Most importantly, do not feel guilty, do not let others make you feel guilty; do not become discouraged. You have no idea how many times I have given in to my cravings. Do I feel bad? No. I looked at each slip as information, as a lesson in what was not working. The next day I tried something different. I have always had the attitude that my life is an experiment in living—healthy eating is no different. The only failure is to quit.

It certainly helps to think about what happened when you do slip up. Think about what you could have done differently. Learn from your mistakes. Understand that while trial and error will eventually get you there, it is not a very efficient way to change. Better to utilize the wisdom of those who have already made the change. That is why I am always reading what others have written about raw food. Besides learning new ideas, it is extremely motivating.

You should also understand that change, radical change as in becoming a raw food person, is more difficult than you expect in the beginning. You have a whole lifetime of being brainwashed to overcome.

Willpower is not enough, you will need all of the processes discussed above and you will need them over and over again.

Termination

A word on termination—don't worry about it. There will come a day when you do not have to think about how you are eating. It will be effortless. I do not know this in the world of raw food, but I do know it from changing other behaviors. Looking back on the changes that I have made in my life I can see the various stages and processes. I went through them without being aware of what I was doing—imagine how much easier it will be when we have a ready-made outline of the course ahead of time.

Personal Transformation

Change is not just a mechanical "do this and this will result" kind of thing. In other words, change is not a science, it is an art. Even more than that, change has a spiritual dimension—it is about personal growth and transformation. When the food that you eat causes less suffering for animals, less destruction of the planet, and more energy and health for you, it is not just your body that benefits. You will become a different person. I think your soul, the essence of who you are, will shine more and you and others will become aware of that.

I did my doctoral dissertation on personal transformation. After a year of research, writing, and reflecting, I discovered a few things about the process of change in human beings. Personal transformation is messy, it is mysterious, and it is multi-dimensional. As much as we like to think we are in control of our lives—we are not.

I found that while we cannot control the processes and events of our lives, we can chose to cooperate with them. We can surrender to the flow of life and the evolutionary forces at work on this planet. Change is chaotic and mysterious, paradoxical and transformational. But there are things that we can do, having more to do with attitude than with action.

We can learn to quiet our minds and become more aware—more aware of what is going on, on a deeper level. We can ask ourselves what is it that we are meant to be learning through this experience. We can surrender to the events and circumstances of our lives, changing what we can, accepting what we can't. We can learn through our suffering. Pain is a wonderful motivator. I find that when I am in pain, I really try harder to be self-aware. All of this points to life and our life experiences as what really changes us. Are we really running our own lives?

The spiritual aspect of change is extremely significant.

"For most gulls, it is not flying that matters, but eating. For this gull, though, it was not eating that mattered, but flight."

–RICHARD BACH, FROM "JONATHAN LIVINGSTON SEAGULL"

For Additional Reading on Change:

Changing for Good: A Revolutionary Six-stage Program for Overcoming Bad Habits and Moving Your Life Positively Forward. Prochaska, James O., Norcross, John C., and Diclemente, Carlo C. (1994). Harper Collins.

Chapter 15

Recipes to Live For

"Once I went raw, I felt, for the first time in my life, completely liberated from food. I just don't think about food the way I used to."

—ALISSA COHEN

Eating healthy foods is not as difficult as you might think. After all, what is so inherently tasty about eating a cheeseburger, or salmon steak, or filet mignon? What makes these foods taste good, while most people do not get all excited about a tomato and romaine salad? We know that we really don't want to know what is in that ground up meat, we don't want to think about how that salmon (which is advertised as Wild Atlantic, but is actually grown in a fish farm near the coast) contains all kinds of antibiotics and parasites, and we certainly don't want to know how that cow was slaughtered and cut up for our consumption.

Eating animal products is not an inherently enjoyable event. We are just accustomed to it. My grandchildren have been raised as vegans and when they want a treat they ask for veggies, smoothies, fruit-based ice cream, nuts, and an assortment of other healthy foods.

From the look on their faces it is obvious that they are enjoying themselves. They would look on in disgust at a grilled sausage. It is only habit and custom that stop us all from eating foods that make us healthy, light, and happy.

The key and essential element to changing our dietary habits, besides education, is to have at our disposal a bunch of great raw food recipes. I am including in this chapter just those that I use for the main part of my diet. These are my all-time favorites because they taste great and are easy to make. The following recipes are a good start, but I suggest several other books at the end of this chapter that I have found particularly helpful. I also strongly suggest using youtube to search for recipes. Seeing is so much better than reading. All of the following recipes can be found on youtube.com and my blog.

Smoothies

Smoothies are the foundation and easy entrance into a world raw vegan delights. Smoothies nourish your body and begin the painless work of introducing your system to living foods. They are the advance army building an information network that will make the smooth transition to a healthy diet.

I offer two basic kinds of smoothies here: my morning green fruit smoothie and my afternoon superfood green smoothie. I often have both in a day. You could start out with one. Mix them up; alternate days. Or have both. Smoothies are the best way to get lots of fruit and green leafy vegetables into your diet without a lot of work.

Green Fruit Smoothie

1	cup liquid (water, coconut water, or tea)
2	oranges freshly squeezed
2	handfuls of goji berries
½	cup pineapple
½	cup frozen strawberries
½	cup frozen wild blueberries
4-5	leaves of romaine, red or green leaf lettuce, kale, or a handful or two of spinach

You can add your favorite fruits and subtract whatever you don't like. Experiment until the smoothie tastes great to you. Put the liquid in the blender first, then the soft fruit, greens, and put the frozen fruit in last. This smoothie makes a great breakfast. I highly suggest investing in a Vita-Mix blender. They are expensive, but you will use them every day, they will last forever, and you will find you can't live without it.

Superfood Green Smoothie

2	cups liquid (water, juice, tea, etc)
3	bananas (one frozen)
1	celery stalk (optional)
4-5	leaves of romaine, kale, collard greens, or Swiss chard
1	TBS raw cacao powder
1	TBS raw agave
1	TBS Spirulina or Blue Green Algae
1	TBS raw coconut butter
½	TSP maca
1	TSP dulse, or nori, or kelp
1	TSP hemp seeds

Put the liquid in first, then the bananas, goji berries, leaves, super foods, and the frozen banana last. The ingredients in this smoothie are not cast in stone either. Experiment until you love the taste. Try other super foods as well. This makes a great lunch to go.

Super Food Smoothie Leather (rollup)

Take the ingredients for the above Super Food Smoothie, except for the water, and blend in a food processor. Pour onto Excalibur Paraflexx non-stick sheets. Then put in a dehydrator for about 24 hours. You now can take it with you on a plane or wherever you want to go. Stores well for days.

Salad Dressings

An arsenal of four or five delicious salad dressings is essential if you are going to have one big salad every day. My recipes all come from my daughter Gina. I don't know what I would have done without her and the dressings. As for the salads themselves, I don't do anything fancy because I don't want to spend the time. I use green or red leaf lettuce, or romaine. I usually throw in some baby spinach greens or arugula.

You can add in whatever else you like: peppers, cucumbers, tomatoes, walnuts, sunflower seeds, ground flaxseeds, etc. An avocado will make the salad very filling.

Gina's Favorite

2	cups olive or flaxseed oil
2	TBS Nama Shoyu or raw soy sauce
2	TBS raw tahini
1	piece of ginger, about 2 inches long
½	cup of lemon juice
6	cloves of garlic

nutritional yeast for flavor (amount depends on your taste)
(warning, too much nutritional yeast can cause headaches)
Put ingredients in blender and enjoy. This is my favorite salad dressing, too.

Sweet Italian Dressing

1	cup olive oil
1	cup raw apple cider vinegar
½	cup raw agave
2	TBS dulse or kelp
	Italian seasonings (optional)

This is my favorite light summer dressing when the weather gets hot.

Creamy Balsamic Vinegar

½	cup tahini
½	cup flaxseed or olive oil
½	cup balsamic vinegar
2	TBS lemon juice
6	cloves garlic
	raw agave to taste (optional)
	raw mustard to taste (optional)

Put ingredients in the blender. Add water to achieve desired consistency. This also makes for a great vegetable dip if served directly from the refrigerator.

Tahini Lemon Dressing

⅔   cup tahini

½   cup lemon juice

¼   cup flaxseed oil

¼   cup water

2   TBS raw agave

1   clove garlic

Put ingredients into the blender. This also makes for a great veggie dip.

Entrees

The following are not really entrees, but that is how I eat them. They are what I have after I've had my smoothies and salads to top things off for the day. These dishes tend to have more nuts and fats, which are better consumed at this time. As a general principle think of having fruits early in the day, then salads, then nuts, seeds, and fats.

Cauliflower Mashed Potatoes

2	cups cauliflower
½	cup cashews
¼	cup olive or flaxseed oil
1	TBS dulse or kelp
1	very small clove of garlic
	black pepper
	dill
	hot pepper sesame oil (optional)

Throw everything into the food processor until it looks like mashed potatoes. This is one of my all-time favorites.

Chicken-Tuna Pretend Salad

1 ½	cups soaked sunflower seeds
1	cup cashews
¾	cup of coconut water (or plain water)
½	cup of lemon juice
2	stalks of celery, diced
2	TBS dulse or kelp
¼	cup dill
2	cloves of garlic
1	TBS thyme
1	TBS oregano
1	TBS sage
1	TBS ground mustard

Place all ingredients in a food processor and mix till done.
You can eat this plain or wrap in romaine leaves.

Marinara Sauce

1	cup fresh tomatoes
1	cup sun dried tomatoes
¼	yellow onion
½	cup lemon juice
3	dates
2	TBS olive or flaxseed oil
2	TBS soy sauce
3	cloves of garlic
1	TBS dulse or kelp

Put all ingredients in a food processor until smooth. This sauce is a staple of my diet. I often mix a couple tablespoons with a mashed up avocado to make a delicious guacamole and have it with my salad for dinner. Or, I put a zucchini through a spiralizer, making raw spaghetti and top it with the marinara sauce.

Dessert

The great thing about raw desserts is that you can eat them anytime and as a replacement for a main meal. They are good for you.

Chocolate Ice Cream and Chocolate Mousse

2	cups durian (a delicious fruit sold in Asian markets)
2	cups cashews
1	cup water
1	cup raw agave
¼	cup coconut butter (or coconut oil, the same thing)
2	TBS vanilla extract
4	TBS raw cacao powder
½	TSP salt or dulse

Put everything in the blender, chill, and then put into an ice cream maker.

After the ice cream is made I add in cacao nibs that taste like chocolate chips and walnuts. Another option is to skip the ice cream step and eat after chilling, this makes for a great mousse. Variations are endless.

Cacao Durian Pudding

2	cups durian
1	cup water
¼	cup pitted dates
2	TBS raw cacao powder

Mix in a blender, chill, and take this with you wherever you go.

The options here are endless. Add in a banana, or strawberries.

My Favorite Raw "Cookbooks"

Living on Live Foods. Alissa Cohen. 2004. Cohen Publishing Company; Kittery, Me.

Raw Food Made Easy for 1 or 2 People. Jennifer Cornbleet. 2005. Book Publishing Company; Summertown, TN.

RAWvolution: Gourmet Living Cuisine. Matt Amsden. 2006. HarperCollins Publishers; New York, NY.

The Raw Revolution Diet. Cherie Soria, Brenda Davis, and Vesanto Melina. 2008. Healthy Living Publications.

Everyday Raw. Mathew Kenney. 2008. Gibbs Smith.

Chapter 16

A Holistic Perspective

"In the seeing of who you are not, the reality of who you are emerges by itself."

—ECKHART TOLLE

Something interesting happens after your diet becomes more alive— you become more alive. Something very interesting and wonderful is going on. I can't speak for everyone, but for many of the people I have met on this journey, I find that this is true. First, you become happier. I look back to how I felt before and how I feel now and I am definitely happier. And it feels as if it comes from the food. Second, you become more peaceful. And third, you connect a bit more with other people.

There is scientific research showing that green leafy vegetables supply the body with lots of absorbable calcium. Besides building strong bones, calcium has a wonderful calming effect on the body. It relieves stress. We all know that chocolate enhances our moods and my superfood smoothies contain plenty of raw cacao powder. It makes sense that when you nourish your body, and when it doesn't feel deprived of what it needs, you will feel happier.

Another aspect of feeling happier, I think, involves the karma (we reap what we sow) of a vegan diet. As our food choices result in fewer animals dying and suffering, we can find pleasure in our eating and enjoy the benefits of creating a better place for all creatures. In addition, our vegan food choices result in less pollution and trashing of our planet. This, too, must at some level come back to us as a sense of living more wholesome, lightly, and happily.

This sense of being happier seems to open people up to more spirituality. If there was no spirituality to begin with, then something new happens. If it was already there, the spirituality seems to deepen. I rarely meet people involved in this raw food journey who do not share a sense of spiritual awakening and deepening. Is it that our bodies are no longer weighted down with dead food particles? Can we see better, can we see more, now that our blood is purer? Is there an unconscious loss of guilt because we are contributing less to the suffering of animals? Whatever it is, it seems to open doors.

So what does this deeper sense of spirituality look like? For me it comes as awareness, awakening, a wider perspective. First, I am more aware of my body. I feel what is happening inside more clearly. I notice my feet and legs, muscle tightness, and the pleasure of stretching them out. I enjoy yoga and feeling my body relax. It is impossible to eat raw vegan foods and be fat. My lighter body is a joy to carry around now. I'm not as self-conscious of its aging.

I am aware of the space inside my body. While I have come to enjoy my body more, I have also come to realize that while I like this body, I am not my body. I have this body, but who I am is something so much larger than this physical living thing that I have always thought was me, all of me. I sense my real self as something beyond my body.

When I look at my body, when I am aware of my body, I also become aware that there is a part of me that is aware, that is observing. So, what is this observing thing? Am I the observer (my true self) or am I the observed (my body)? And this observing self, if it is not in the body, where is it? It feels like it is everywhere. It feels like it never aged. It feels like the little boy who loved making sandcastles at the beach and still wants to be where the ocean makes love to the seashore endlessly.

This sense of awareness extends to my mind and my thoughts. Who thinks about thoughts? I'm hungry, I eat. Now, I'm hungry and I think. Something upsets me, and I become aware instead of just reacting. Oh, that old woman in that car is going so slowly, and I'm in such a hurry. Why am I in a hurry? Why am I driving so close to her? Do I really want to make her nervous? I am aware of my life and my thoughts. I love it. Instead of just being driven by what happens outside of me, I now have choices. I don't have to become sad because I am by myself today. I can choose to enjoy the beauty of my world. I can do this because I am aware of my thoughts.

If I am aware of my thoughts, then I must not be my thoughts. Here we go again. So who am I? I have thoughts, but I am not my thoughts. I am the thinker of my thoughts. I can choose to have other thoughts. Even better, I can choose not to have any thoughts and just enjoy life as it is. Awareness of my thoughts is one of the most powerful skills I have ever been given.

This raw vegan approach to life has helped me become more aware of my body, my mind, and the spiritual aspect of my life as well. But this is where it gets interesting. I am aware of my body and my thoughts, but when it comes to my spirituality, that does not feel accurate. It feels like our spirituality. I am not aware of my spirituality because maybe there is no "my spirituality," there is only "our" spirituality. And this points to seeing the essence of spirituality itself. Is it that the "I" who we usually refer to as ourselves may not really be there at all? Maybe there is only "we" and no "I."

When I become aware of my body and how I am not my body, the observer in me does not feel like an isolated individual but a connected being, connected to everything in the universe. It is the same with the thinker of my thoughts. That thinker does not feel singular but infinite. There is a transcendence going on.

So, how can one not be happy to discover all of this? This renewed sense of spirituality is about being connected. I feel connected to this planet, this universe, the plants, animals, sunsets. I feel connected to my neighbors, here and on the other side of the world. My family has no bounds. My life has no bounds. Awareness for me has become a discovery that happiness comes from being a part of all that is, accepting all that is, loving all that is.

Happiness is not a destination, it is a journey. I am not a one hundred percent raw vegan person. Maybe I never will be. That is okay because

I am on the journey, just like you. I will make mistakes and will forget who I am. I am sure I will have ice cream now and again, although my durian ice cream is exceptionally good. But life is a journey, that is where the fun is. Let's not be too hard on ourselves. We learn by mistakes. That is what forgiveness is for. Don't worry, be reasonable, rational, and realistically raw.

For Additional Readings on Holistic Perspectives:

Holistic Perspectives & Integral Theory: On Seeing What Is. Frank Ferendo, Ph.D. 2007. Process Publishing Company.

A New Earth: Awakening to Your Life's Purpose. Eckhart Tolle. 2005. Penguin Group.

Breinigsville, PA USA
31 December 2009
229981BV00003B/26/P

9 780979 518027